Advance praise for *The TMJ Healing Plan*

"This is the most useful book of its kind that has ever been written and should be required reading for all TMD patients, dentists who treat TMD, and physicians who see patients who might have TMD. I will definitely have my Orofacial Pain residents at UCLA read this book and have several copies available in my office. When given appropriate professional care...patients who use this book to eliminate harmful habits and implement appropriate home-care activities will have the best chance for a speedy and thorough return to normal function."

— Joseph R. Cohen, DDS, FACD,
President, American Board of Orofacial Pain,
Adjunct Asst. Professor, UCLA Orofacial Pain,
TMD, and Sleep Apnea Residency Program

"This book is loaded with nuggets of information that can help patients help themselves. Cynthia Peterson has placed a lifetime of experiences into a guide to help not only TMJ disorders, but other common pain complaints. If you have face pain, this book will offer relief."

— Jeffrey P. Okeson, DMD,
Provost's Distinguished Service Professor
Professor and Chair, Department of Oral Health Science,
Director, Orofacial Pain Program, University of Kentucky College of Dentistry

"What a fantastic resource for health-care providers and patients and for those with and even without TMD!... As a rheumatologist, I was pleased with Cynthia's evidence-based approach, focusing on a patient's proactive role in performing exercises and addressing underlying causes instead of encouraging expensive unproved therapies.... The pertinent anecdotes, practical solutions, and inherent encouragement in this book will be of great value to many patients."

— Stephanie Boade Silas, MD

"This book explains the causes of TMJ, its symptoms, and most importantly, the nonsurgical treatments available to deal with it. I've had TMJ most of my adult life, and I found it was getting worse not better as time progressed. The surgical approaches I'd researched sounded too radical, and nothing else was working. This book ... when followed, will start you on the road to recovery. I started seeing an improvement with my TMJ condition within a few days."

— Jon Howard

"A key turning point in the treatment of my TMJ disorder came when I attended Cynthia Peterson's "Jaw School." She enabled me to see a much-clearer picture of what aggravates my jaw and neck trouble, and more importantly what I can do to promote healing and freedom from pain. I saw the most improvement after utilizing her instruction. I'm grateful to now have Cynthia's knowledge and expertise in book form. Her style is pleasant and the information easy to grasp. I will refer to her book often when I have questions or need a reminder of the principles that keep TMJ problems in check. I highly recommend this book to anyone needing practical, effective solutions to jaw, neck, and headache pain."

— Sara Robinson

"I have lectured to and taught thousands of orthodontists in the U.S., Canada, and around the world, and we all have a common need for a publication that educates patients. A high percentage of people in the U.S. and Canada suffer from varying degrees of TMJ disorders.... This book addresses all aspects of the disorder, including prevention, that I would want to share with my patients."

— Randall K. Bennett DDS, MS

"Cynthia: I have read through your book with interest and feel that it presents an excellent program of self-management for TMD patients. Commonly, patients with TMD pain don't know what they can do to decrease their pain and also don't understand what they have been doing that may have influenced the development of their pain. I would unhesitatingly recommend this book to those suffering from TM disorders. I look forward to its publication."

— Robert L. Merrill, DDS, MS,
Adjunct Professor, Director, Orofacial Pain and
Dental Sleep Medicine Center, UCLA School of Dentistry

"This book offers a clear and concise explanation of a very complex problem. It is a valuable resource that I will recommend to all of my patients who suffer from TMJ disorders."

— Reid Swenson, Orthodontist

The
TMJ Healing Plan

TEN STEPS TO RELIEVING

HEADACHES, NECK PAIN

AND JAW DISORDERS

Cynthia Peterson, PT

Foreword by James L. Guinn, DMD

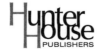

Hunter House
PUBLISHERS

Hunter House Inc., Publishers
PO Box 2914
Alameda CA 94501-0914

Illustration and photo credits are located on page vi

Library of Congress Cataloging-in-Publication Data
Peterson, Cynthia.
The TMJ healing plan : 10 steps to relieving headaches, neck pain and jaw disorders / Cynthia Peterson. — 1st ed.
p. cm.—(Positive options for health series)
Includes bibliographical references and index.
ISBN 978-0-89793-524-1 (pbk. : alk. paper)   1. Temporomandibular joint—Diseases—Exercise therapy.   I. Title.
RK470.P48 2009
617.5'220642—dc22   2009024791

Project Credits
Cover Design: Stefanie Gold Design   Illustrations: Jennifer Peterson
Photographers: Lara Gallagher, Clara Thorup, and Karen Harrop
Models: Sunny Harvey, Lara Gallagher, Lincoln Taylor, Sarah Edwards,
Jodi Nichols, Kathryn Gwynn, and Aticus Peterson
Book Production: John McKercher   Senior Marketing Associate: Reina Santana
Developmental Editor: Jude Berman   Publicity Coordinator: Sean Harvey
Copy Editor: Mary Miller   Rights Coordinator: Candace Groskreutz
Proofreader: John David Marion   Order Fulfillment: Washul Lakdhon
Indexer: Cynthia Peterson   Administrator: Theresa Nelson
Managing Editor: Alexandra Mummery   Computer Support: Peter Eichelberger
Customer Service Manager: Christina Sverdrup
Publisher: Kiran S. Rana

Printed and bound by Sheridan Books, Ann Arbor, Michigan
Manufactured in the United States of America

9 8 7 6 5 4 3 2 1   First Edition   10 11 12 13 14

DEDICATION

This book is dedicated to my beloved children,
Aticus, Anna Caroline, and Amadeus.
May you use whatever time, talents, and abundance
God has blessed you with to bless the lives of others.

This book is also my gift to each of you
for a healthier, happier life.

Ordering

Trade bookstores in the U.S. and Canada please contact:

Publishers Group West
1700 Fourth Street, Berkeley CA 94710
Phone: (800) 788-3123   Fax: (800) 351-5073

Hunter House books are available at bulk discounts for textbook course adoptions; to qualifying community, health-care, and government organizations; and for special promotions and fund-raising.
For details please contact:

Special Sales Department
Hunter House Inc., PO Box 2914, Alameda CA 94501-0914
Phone: (510) 865-5282   Fax: (510) 865-4295
E-mail: ordering@hunterhouse.com

Individuals can order our books from most bookstores, by calling **(800) 266-5592**, or from our website at
www.hunterhouse.com

Contents

Foreword by James L. Guinn, DMD x

Preface xii

Acknowledgments xv

Introduction 1

    What Is TMJ? 1

    Who Should Read This Book? 2

    How Do You Know If You Have a TMJ Disorder? 2

    How to Use This Book 4

1 Replacing Hurtful Habits 7

    From Hurtful to Healthy 7

    The 10 Steps 8

2 Important Anatomy 10

    The Temporomandibular Joints 10

    PoTSB TLC 17

    Summary 18

3 Step 1: Stop the Overuse and Abuse of Your Jaw 19

    When Your Joints Break Down 19

    What You Can Do to Slow Down Wear and Tear 23

    Summary 27

4 Step 2: The Power of Posture: Learn How to Stand,
Sit, and Sleep 29

    Why You Want Good Posture 29

    How to Assess Your Posture 33

Seeking Professional Help for Postural Problems 35
Put Perfect Posture into Practice: How to Stand 40
Put Perfect Posture into Practice: How to Sit 47
Put Perfect Posture into Practice: How to Sleep 55
Summary 64

5   Step 3: TLC: Teeth Apart, Lips Together,
    and Calm Your Muscles and Mind. 67
The Harm of Teeth Touching 67
Bracing, Clenching, and Grinding 68
What You Can Do to Stop Bracing, Clenching,
    and Grinding 70
Retraining for TLC: Teeth Apart, Lips Together, and
    Calm Muscles and Mind. 77
Summary 81

6   Step 4: Train Your Tongue and
    Swallow Carefully 83
The Resting Position of the Mandible 84
Tongue on the Roof 84
Swallow Correctly 93
Still Having Trouble? 102
Summary 103

7   Step 5: Breathe Well 105
Running Out of Gas 105
Chest Breathing Is Breathing Turned Upside Down 106
The Obstacles to Breathing Your Best 108
Assess How You Breathe 111
What You Can Do to Breathe Well 113
Seek Professional Help 118
Summary 118

8   Step 6: Care for Your Muscles 120
Myofascial Pain 120
Restore and Maintain a Full Range of Motion 131

Fibromyalgia 164
Summary 167

9 Step 7: Care for Your Disks and
Ligamentous Structures 169
Disks 170
Joints, Ligaments, and Hypermobility 179
Summary 182

10 Step 8: Halt Head and Neck Pain 184
Headaches 185
Neck Pain 190
First Aid When You Need It 192
Summary 196

11 Step 9: Reduce Stress and Begin to Exercise 198
Fight-or-Flight Versus Rest-and-Digest 198
What You Can Do to Reduce Stress 201
Regular Exercise: A Cycle of Success 205
Start Your Exercise Program 209
Summary 218

12 Step 10: Make Your Action Plan 220
What Do You Want to Change? 220
Choosing a Provider and Seeing a Specialist 225
A Plea to Parents and Health-Care Professionals
Working with Children and Young Adults 226
Conclusion 228

Resources 229
Notes 231
References 246
Index 258

Foreword

There may be no other clinical condition as misunderstood, misdiagnosed, and mistreated as jaw disorders and associated pain. Patients seeking help for these problems can easily be led to believe their problem is due to a particular cause, when the truth may lie elsewhere. This can occur whether the patient is seeking help on the Internet, through books, or during a consultation with a doctor. Too often, the person claiming to have knowledge about these problems has a bias or hidden agenda. Following the recommendations of such a person can lead to unnecessary (and expensive) treatment.

The average patient with a jaw disorder has seen several different doctors, most of whom had divergent opinions, and is still seeking relief after undergoing a variety of failed treatments. Often, friends and family members do not understand the pain and misery patients are enduring, because they look "normal." Too many patients with these problems are dismissed by their doctors as being "just stressed out."

To be fair, jaw disorders can be very challenging to diagnose and manage. This is true partly because two different patients with similar complaints can have totally different underlying conditions. Trying to apply the same treatment regimen to both patients can result in at least one of them receiving no significant benefit. Unless the cause (or usually the combination of several causes) is identified, a treatment plan with predictable results cannot be made.

While there may not be "easy" answers for patients with these problems, there are answers. This book goes a long way in providing those answers, but it does not advocate a "one-size-fits-all" or "cookbook" approach to treatment. What it does do is provide a wealth of information about the components of jaw disorders and the many ways harmful habits or poor lifestyle choices can lead to a constellation of symptoms in the head, jaw, and neck. Thus, patients can identify potential causes for their particular condition, along with reasonable treatment options.

For patients with a jaw disorder, this book is an oasis in a desert of confusion, misinformation, and marketing hype. It is well researched and based on the best-available evidence at the present time. The recommendations provided here are conservative. Following these guidelines can certainly help but not hurt the patient. However, as the author points out, this book is not a substitute for a thorough evaluation by a qualified clinician, should your symptoms persist. There are obviously certain problems within this field (such as arthritis in the jaw) that patients cannot evaluate or treat themselves. While conservative management is always best, there can be underlying problems, which require specialized care and consideration using sound clinical judgment and evidence-based medical resources.

This book is appropriate for those seeking self-help options, as well as for those currently under the care of a clinician. It is a very good educational text on the anatomy and function of the jaw and related structures. Following the guidelines in this book can also help prevent a recurrence of jaw problems in the future.

Physical therapist Cynthia Peterson has been a great help to my patients for many years, as they have attended her excellent classes on jaw disorders. She has dedicated her professional life to educating and empowering patients. With this well-written resource book, many more people can have access to her knowledge, expertise, and insights. It will be a valuable guide for patients and an effective tool for clinicians treating these problems. It provides a wealth of well-documented techniques for relief of jaw symptoms.

It is my sincere hope that the clear and concise information in this book can provide answers for those suffering from chronic pain in and around the jaw. This book is written by someone who truly understands the nature and complexity of jaw disorders, as well as the impact these problems can have on a person's quality of life.

— James L. Guinn, DMD
Diplomate, American Board of Orofacial Pain

Preface

Years ago, I was diagnosed with an early breast cancer and underwent several major surgeries; before that, I lost my talented mother-in-law, who left a legacy of art that touches many lives, to cancer. As a result of these encounters with illness, I took a fresh look at my life to reassess how I might make a difference in the world. I am not an artist, although my bubble letters and suns are pretty good. Of course, my children and family were my first thought and priority. However, I wondered if I could leave any additional legacy.

This book is one answer to that question. I love being a physical therapist and empowering people, especially those who have TMJ-related disorders, with the education, tools, and exercises they need to become healthy and active again. I love being a detective of the body and deciphering why my patients are having problems.

When I first started teaching my patients about the jaw, neck, and back, I felt I was sharing hidden truths they badly needed but didn't have access to. My heart still aches each time I meet a twelve-or thirteen-year-old who has already destroyed his or her jaw joints. Unfortunately, people usually don't have a desire to learn and change until they find themselves in serious pain or experience a loss of function. Maybe for this reason, healthy habits rarely become a topic of conversation around the dinner table. But they should be.

After years of working with patients who suffered from head, neck, and jaw pain, I decided it was time to write this book. In my work and in this book, I offer an important supplement to the traditional medical model. That model primarily throws a pill or slaps a bandage at the problem, instead of digging deep and addressing the causes and contributing factors. Patients, too, demand a quick fix, rather than seeking to make the changes necessary for long-term relief. However, I believe we all need to find and eliminate the causes of our problems and not just treat the symptoms. As Thomas Edison once said, "The doctor of the future will give no medicine, but will interest his patients in the care of the human frame, in diet and in the cause and prevention of disease."

Imagine a walkway in front of your home that is full of bumps, gaps, and holes. You must traverse this path every day, and yet you frequently trip, slip, or fall into a hole. If the sidewalk is never repaired, you are likely to be hurt over and over again. Similarly, you and your health-care providers must find and patch as many holes as possible in your life's pathways by correcting the causes or contributing factors you may unknowingly be falling into, so you are not doomed to "endless cycles of treatment and relapses."[1] In this book, I offer information that can help you patch many of your own holes. No two people are the same; thus it is up to you to decide with your health-care providers which of the concepts I present that you wish to embrace. I focus on several hurtful habits that are possible causes or contributing factors for problems common to the TMJ population. I offer conservative and reversible ways to replace them with healthier habits.

My colleagues at Canyon Rim Physical Therapy and I have more than fifty years of combined experience in treating patients with a wide range of TMJ-related symptoms and problems and educating this patient population, with much clinical success. It often takes a team of dedicated professionals from all areas of the medical arena to ensure the whole patient is treated. In writing this book, I have sought out experts and incorporated the wisdom from multiple disciplines to create a multifaceted approach. This book gives you the basics for each specialty area addressed and at the same time provides the convenience of having all of the topics presented in one volume. My aim is to educate you on the basics and then point you in the right direction if more help is needed. This book introduces you to ideas and principles that are often overlooked in even the most clearly presented cases. I combine everything with some good old common sense and an occasional dose of humor. I also include stories and examples of patients throughout (to protect their privacy and for the purpose of brevity, I have changed names and any identifying information).

Much more research and awareness is needed to improve the lives of those suffering from TMJ-related disorders. I will donate 10 percent of the royalties I receive from this book to support TMJ-related research and awareness.

Most of all, I want to help people like you. This book is my gift to you for a healthier, happier life. May you and yours be blessed with all the wonderful things in life that money can't buy…such as health, love, and the kind of happiness that can only come back to you when you give it away.

Acknowledgments

This book would not have been possible without the unconditional support of my wonderful husband, Bruce, who helped me keep going whenever I felt overwhelmed or discouraged, my talented sister-in-law, Jenny Peterson, who helped with the illustrations and photos, and my dear father, Gary Sandquist. I am indebted and eternally grateful for all of my family, extended family, and God's kindness in prompting me to write this book and opening doors and hearts along the way.

I learned most of what I know about TMJ disorders from my physical therapy mentor and TMJ disorders expert, Steve Shupe, MS, PT, OCS; the owner of Canyon Rim Physical Therapy and one of the most clinically brilliant physical therapists I know. I also want to thank physical therapists Dede Lewis, Wendy Zeigler, Connie Thomsen, and Stacey Corrado. I have had the privilege of knowing and learning from dentist and TMJ expert Dr. James L. Guinn, who has dedicated his professional career and thirty years of his life exclusively to TMJ disorders. He treats patients from four states, and over 600 doctors look to him to help their patients. I am indebted to speech-language pathologist Hilary Wilson, who is specially trained in tongue thrust and swallowing disorders and who made sure my tongue and swallowing chapters were accurate.

Thank you to my fabulous photographers, Lara Gallagher, Clara Thorup, and Karen Harrop, and my marvelous models, Sunny Harvey, Lara Gallagher, Jodi Nichols, Lincoln Taylor, Sarah Edwards, Kathryn Gwynn, and Aticus Peterson. I have relied heavily on the work of many experts who have devoted their entire lives to TMJ and myofascial pain disorders. They are my professional heroes and include world-renowned TMJ experts Dr. Mariano Rocabado, Dr. Jeff Okeson, Dr. Jeff Cohen, and Dr. Jocelyne Feine, many of whom kindly reviewed my materials, the late Dr. Janet Travell, and Dr. David Simons. They also include physical therapists Steven Kraus and Annette Iglarsh. I was guided by the work of talented ergonomists Alan Hedge and Don Bloswick.

I am appreciative of and impressed with Terrie Cowley, National TMJ Association President, who tirelessly serves this patient population and communicated with me on several occasions, and with Milton and Renee Glass, Jaw Joints & Allied Musculo-Skeletal Disorders Foundation (JJAMD) founders, who unselfishly devote their time and efforts to jaw joint disorders and were instrumental in having November named as Jaw Joint/TMJ Awareness Month®. Last, but never least, I have loved working with my capable and talented editors and Hunter House staff Alex Mummery, Jude Berman, Mary Miller, John David Marion, Barbara Moulton, and Kiran Rana.

Important Note

The material in this book is intended to provide a review of resources and information related to temporomandibular joint disorders. Every effort has been made to provide accurate and dependable information. However, professionals in the field may have differing opinions, and change is always taking place. Any of the self-management techniques described herein do not replace a thorough evaluation and should be undertaken only under the guidance of a licensed healthcare practitioner. The author, editors, and publishers cannot be held responsible for any error, omission, professional disagreement, outdated material, or adverse outcomes that derive from use of any of these treatments or information resources in this book, either in a program of self-care or under the care of a licensed practitioner. The author and publisher advise that you check with your physician or licensed health-care provider before starting any exercise, stretching, or self-management program.

Introduction

Before we begin this journey, it is important that you have a basic understanding of what "TMJ" disorders are and some of the symptoms most commonly associated with them.

What Is TMJ?

TMJ is an acronym for the temporomandibular joint, which are the small joints located just in front of each ear. The TMJs are located where the ball-shaped end of your lower jawbone comes in contact with your skull. The lower jawbone, or *mandible,* is attached to the skull on each side by ligaments, muscles, and connective tissue. These two joints are used over a thousand times a day and make it possible for you to talk, eat, chew, swallow, sing, kiss, and make facial expressions. You even use these important joints when you sleep, because you swallow saliva throughout the night. (See Chapter 2 for a discussion of the anatomy of the temporomandibular joint.)

When people have pain or problems involving their temporomandibular joints, they often say, "I have TMJ"; however, that is like someone with ankle problems saying, "I have ankle." Disorders involving the temporomandibular joints and the adjoining muscles and tissues have many names, including TMD (temporomandibular disorders), TMJD (temporomandibular joint disorders), CMD (craniomandibular disorders), or craniofacial pain and OFP (orofacial pain). In this book, I keep it simple and use the term *TMJ disorders* because it is more easily recognized, although in most medical circles, TMD would be the most common acronym used. The lack of consensus even about what to call this disorder makes research difficult and illustrates the confusion people suffering from TMJ-related problems face. Sufferers are left to sort through the confusion and are often not sure where to turn for help. The TMJ Association's report to the National Institutes of Health (NIH) states that "TMD patients see on average 6.9 specialists before receiving a definitive diagnosis. Others, like actor Burt Reynolds, see [as many as] 13."[2]

According to a recent study in the *New England Journal of Medicine*, 40 to 75 percent of adults in the United States report at least one sign of temporomandibular disorders. TMJ disorders are most commonly reported in twenty- to fifty-year-olds. Both men and women experience TMJ problems; however, three to nine times more women than men seek treatment.[3]

The social impact of TMJ-related symptoms is alarming. An estimated $30 billion a year are lost in productivity, along with 550 million lost workdays due to symptoms commonly associated with TMJ, such as headaches and facial pain.[4] Other symptoms can include pain in the jaw joint and surrounding area (including the ear); the jaw locking open or closed; and neck, shoulder, and upper-back pain.

Who Should Read This Book?

If you have a head, neck, and jaw and like to eat, chew, swallow, sing, and talk without pain, then you should benefit from developing the healthy habits outlined in this book. The National Institute for Craniofacial Research (NIDCR) has instituted a "Less Is Often Best in Treating TMJ Disorders" campaign.[5] According to the NIDCR, "Until there is science-based evidence to help health-care providers make sound treatment decisions, NIDCR suggests the following:

1. Try simple self-care practices.

2. Avoid treatments that cause permanent changes to the bite or jaw.

3. Avoid, whenever possible, surgical treatment for TMJ.

This book is full of simple self-care practices and information.

How Do You Know If You Have a TMJ Disorder?

Some people live with a TMJ disorder for years before it becomes painful enough to cause them to seek help. For others, the problem arises suddenly. Nevertheless, both types of people can have very similar symptoms. Others may have jaw joint problems and no pain. People with TMJ disorders seldom have the same complaints and often have multiple symptoms, which can include:

- facial pain and/or swelling
- headaches
- pain or discomfort in the jaw joint and the surrounding areas
- pain, catching, or difficulty opening or closing the mouth
- clicking or grating sounds in the jaws
- locking of the jaw, either open or closed
- ear pain, stuffiness, or ringing in the ears, with no infection present
- neck, shoulder, or upper-back pain
- difficulty in chewing, talking, or yawning
- unbalanced mouth opening or bite problems
- unexplained tooth pain in a healthy tooth
- tooth grinding or clenching
- morning jaw pain or fatigue
- difficulty swallowing

If you have multiple painful joints, you should be evaluated by a rheumatologist who studies joint diseases to ensure you don't have any underlying problems.

TMJ disorders are classified by the National Institutes of Health into the following categories. Many people experience symptoms from more than one or all three of these categories. I have simplified the terminology.

1. **Muscle pain and dysfunction**, or other problems with the muscles and tissues of the jaw and surrounding areas. This is the most common category.

2. **Structural or internal problems,** which means that structures inside the joint are damaged, out of balance, or not working

correctly. Symptoms can include clicking, grinding, crepitus (grating), and locking.

3. **Arthritis and degenerative inflammatory joint disorders** affecting the jaw joints, including osteoarthritis, rheumatoid arthritis, and fibromyalgia.

How to Use This Book

If you are at home and the smoke alarm goes off, what do you do? To do nothing is to risk tragedy. You would immediately investigate what triggered the alarm. Does the battery need to be changed in the smoke alarm or did you leave a roast in the oven and the kitchen is in flames? All too often, our body's alarms go off daily and we ignore them.

For example, after a late night you wake up in the morning on your stomach with your teeth clenched and one arm over your head, and you have a tension headache and a stiff jaw. Ignoring these alarms, you take two painkillers and sit down to a breakfast of chewy bagels and crunchy raw apples. After a quick shower, you grab a cup of coffee or your favorite cola and your 20-pound briefcase, purse, and/or child. Then you run out the door.

Maneuvering through morning traffic makes you tense; then you arrive at work, where the pain in your head, neck, or jaw gets worse. You slouch at your desk, holding the phone to your ear with your shoulder, while you simultaneously listen politely to a customer's complaints and finish typing a presentation. You chew on ice, chew on gum, and drink your third diet cola. You check your e-mail, with your keyboard and mouse at an uncomfortable angle. The stress and pain mount throughout the day, and all the while you wonder why your head, neck, and jaw hurt—never pausing to listen to your body's smoke alarms or investigate why they are going off.

It may not be possible to provide a permanent cure for problems of the head, neck, and jaw. However, by applying the principles in this book, you can learn what perpetuates and even causes many of your body's head, neck, and TMJ alarms. Many causes are under your control and can be overcome.

As you can see from this example, many hurtful habits can irritate your head, neck, and jaw. Thankfully, there are some simple, safe solutions for many of the irritants and problems plaguing those suffering from jaw, head, and neck pain. Smart people like you are more interested than ever in being actively involved in their health care. If you want to take charge of your health, this book can help you do the following:

- Eliminate hurtful habits and replace them with healthy ones.

- Prevent or slow irreversible damage to the jaw joints by addressing irritants.

- Increase awareness and understanding, which leads to increased compliance and better results. For example, a person with a tongue thrust that causes an overbite that then requires braces will certainly fare better if the tongue thrust can be eliminated. Or, a person with a locked jaw due to an overstretched ligament that requires surgery will certainly have better surgical results if she learns the ways the connecting bands became overstretched in the first place and how to change those hurtful habits.

- Employ conservative and reversible treatments. According to a 2008 report in the *New England Journal of Medicine*, 85 to 90 percent of people with a TMJ disorder can be treated with "noninvasive, nonsurgical, and reversible interventions."[6] The NIH pamphlet on TMJ disorders states, "experts strongly recommend using the most conservative, reversible treatments possible."[7] The treatments discussed in this book are both conservative and reversible and can benefit the general public as well as those suffering from specific TMJ symptoms.

- Decrease pain and dysfunction by learning to problem solve and self-manage many of your symptoms.

- Save money. TMJ disorders can be very costly. This book is a very cost-effective and smart way to start. If good habits are established, they can reduce the need for more costly treatments. If other treatments are necessary, the concepts in this book set the stage for more successful outcomes with that treatment.

- Better understand medical terms and anatomy so that you can better understand reports and do meaningful searches on Medline and other reliable sources of information to help plan and coordinate your recovery.

- Be empowered to take charge of your health by keeping a symptom diary so you can start to recognize patterns and so you and your providers can "patch the holes" you may unknowingly keep falling into.

- Communicate more effectively with your health-care professionals.

- Bring disciplines together as a team, enabling coordinated treatment of yourself as a whole.

Putting the ideas from this book to work in your own life can help you find relief from painful symptoms and harmful habits. The suggestions you'll read about are simple and have helped hundreds of other people. I encourage you to work together with your doctor, dentist, and other health-care providers to create the individualized plan that will work best for you. Now let's get started.

1

Replacing Hurtful Habits

As you become aware of hurtful habits and their harmful consequences, you will be more willing to take the next steps and make a concerted effort to replace those hurtful habits with healthy ones. It *will* take some effort. Ideally, you could effortlessly pop a pill or push a button. We all get just one body, and since we cannot trade in our current body for a new one every 50,000 miles, you will be wise to take care of the only one you have. You are worth the investment.

From Hurtful to Healthy

The best way to change or remove a hurtful habit is to replace it with a healthy one. However, most of my patients don't even know that they are doing something that is hurtful to themselves. Reading this book is the first step, because it introduces you to the most common hurtful habits associated with TMJ disorders. As you read this book and become more aware, you can make a list of your specific hurtful habits and develop ideas on how to replace them with healthy ones. You can use Table 1.1 on the next page as a template. The "Checklist for Change" part of the table will make more sense as you read on.

You must also become aware of many of the subconscious things you are doing—things you do all the time without even thinking about them—that may be contributing to your symptoms. You must make posture, breathing, tongue and teeth position, and swallowing all conscious activities. Because habits come from doing the same thing over and over, you have to make yourself consciously go in

Table 1.1: Turning Hurtful into Healthy

HURTFUL HABIT	HEALTHY HABIT	CHECKLIST FOR CHANGE
I sleep on my stomach.	I will sleep on my back or side.	I will put a pillow under or between my knees when I sleep.
		I will place a pillow under my upper arm, use a body pillow, or sew a ball into the front of my pajamas to prevent me from rolling onto my stomach.
		I will tell my partner or spouse to wake me up if I sleep on my stomach.
I slouch when sitting.	I will sit correctly.	I need to adjust both the back of my computer chair and its arm supports.
		I will put a footstool under my desk.
		I will use back supports attached to my car seat.
		I will bring an inflatable back support when traveling.
		I will set my watch alarm to go off every hour during the day for two weeks to remind me to maintain a healthy posture.

the new direction until it becomes automatic. Then you must continue practicing the new habits until you perform them right consistently without even thinking about it. Only then can your healthy habit begin to operate subconsciously. For example, if you have been swallowing or breathing incorrectly for years, it will be easy for you to slip back into hurtful habits. So, to catch yourself from reverting to hurtful habits, you must be diligent. Review your action plan of healthy habits, which you will make at the end of this book. At first you should review it daily and weekly to learn and practice your new healthy habits, and eventually you can move on reviewing it monthly. Reassess whenever you have setbacks to determine which bad habits have crept back into your daily life.

The 10 Steps

This book presents a 10-step process. The steps do not have to be followed in any specific order; however, some steps do support each other. For example, healthy posture can make several of the helpful habits easier to achieve. Also, achieving the correct tongue position and strength can make it easier to swallow correctly. You will want to prioritize based on what activities you do most and that have the greatest impact on you. For example, you sleep in the same position for approximately eight hours at a time, so this is typically a *very* important step to fix early on. Also, if your symptoms are reproduced every time you swallow incorrectly, then addressing swallowing will be a top priority.

As you read each step, please **take notes**. Write down the habits you need to change and the ideas you feel will be the most helpful in your situation. (If you own this book, you may even want to write in the margins.) When you reach Step 10, you will pull these notes together to create your own action plan. Later, when you assess how well your plan is working, you can save time by looking at your notes and reminding yourself of the most important points for you.

As you identify the habits you need to replace, **decide to make the necessary changes right at that moment**. For example, after reading about posture in sitting, find a back support and attach it to your chair. When you learn about the ideal sleeping positions, set up your pillows correctly right after reading about it. Other habits will require reminders.

Please use this book actively. Apply the suggestions I have made to your own unique situation, using the help of appropriate healthcare professionals, if necessary. Every person's body and situation is different. If you come up with other ideas or suggestions, send them my way. I would love to share them with others who might also find them helpful. You can contact me through my website at www.tmj healingplan.com.

2

Important Anatomy

Knowledge is power, so it is important for you to begin with a working knowledge of how the temporomandibular joint functions and is put together. This will help you understand what factors may contribute to dysfunction and pain. You'll better understand how the exercises and other suggestions made in the 10 steps that follow can help you.

The Temporomandibular Joints

The temporomandibular joints connect the lower jaw, or mandible, to the sides of your head, or temporal bones. Thus, they are called the *temporo-mandibular joints,* or the joints where these two bones come together (see Figure 2.1). There are two temporomandibular joints, one on either side. They are located very close to your ears. In fact, you can usually feel your temporomandibular joints move by gently placing your fingers in the opening of your ears and opening and closing your mouth. I think this is easiest to feel with your palms forward so that the soft pads of your fingers are facing the joint. The TMJs are somewhat like loose, flexible door hinges. They swing open like a door; however, they also glide or slide forward as you open your mouth. There are several components of the TMJs.

Temporal Bone

The temporal bone is the part of the skull on the sides of your head just above and around your ears. This area of your face is commonly

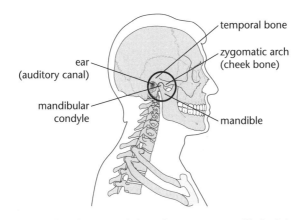

FIGURE 2.1: Skull with a view of the right temporomandibular joint (TMJ)

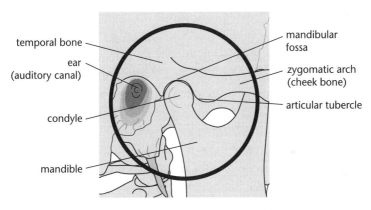

FIGURE 2.2: A closer look at the right temporomandibular joint (TMJ)

referred to as your temples and includes a part of your cheekbones called the *zygomatic arch*. There are rounded notches in the temporal bone called the mandibular fossa (see Figure 2.2). The fossa is the groove where the ball, or condyle, on top of the lower mandible connects and rotates with the temporal bone on each side of the head. In front of the groove, or fossa, is a bump called the *articular tubercle* that helps keep the condyle from gliding too far forward. The ear canal, or *auditory meatus*, is located in the temporal bone and is very close to the temporomandibular joints. This proximity helps explain why some TMJ symptoms include ear symptoms, such as pain, ringing in the ears, stuffy ears, and pressure.

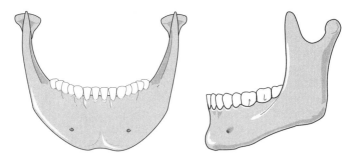

FIGURE 2.3: Front and side view of the mandible, or lower jaw

Mandible and Mandibular Condyle

Your lower jawbone is called the *mandible*. At the top of each side of the lower jaw bone, or mandible, is a ball-shaped bump called your *mandibular condyle* (see Figure 2.3). Some patients are born with abnormally shaped condyles, or they suffer from other problematic anatomical features that predispose them to TMJ problems. When patients have pictures taken of their TMJ and are told they have, for example, worn away 50 percent of their bone, the bone the doctor is typically referring to the ball-shaped condyle. Bones in the body are not designed to rub against each other. The point where the ball-shaped bone on top of the mandible articulates with, or moves against, the temporal bone is not an exception. Wearing down bones can really hurt. When bones rub together, the irritation can cause osteoarthritis. Bone spurs can develop, making the joint bumpy instead of smooth. Typically, grinding and crepitus, which sounds like tires crackling on gravel, are signs of wear and tear in the joint. Special equipment is sometimes necessary to detect very fine crepitus or grinding.

When the joint is irritated, it can cause or increase muscle soreness and tension, which further irritates the joint, creating a painful cycle. If you have arthritis or inflammatory problems throughout your body, such as rheumatoid arthritis, this process of degeneration tends to occur more quickly.

There is a fundamental feature of bone commonly called Wolff's Law. This law explains how cells respond to mechanical stimuli like movement and pressure. Its fundamental concept is that you need the right amount of healthy movement and stress to make your bones and associated structures stronger.[1] This is why people who are prone to osteoporosis, or weakening of their bones, are told to exercise. Too little stress and movement can make the bones so thin that they resorb and become weak.

However, because we use our jaw joints so frequently, the problem is usually too much stress and abnormal movement, which can make the bones bumpy or cause them to wear down in an unhealthy way.

Unfortunately, I have seen a surprising number of teenagers who have advanced osteoarthritis and have already worn away 50 to 60 percent of the ball-shaped mandibular condyle. Because many of your joints tend to deteriorate over time, it behooves you to take good care of all your joints, including your jaw joints. If you don't, you may risk putting your ability to eat, talk, and swallow in jeopardy. In Chapter 3, I will discuss ways you can practice healthy movement and protect your jaw joints to help slow down this degenerative process.

Articular Disk

The articular disk is a dense, fibrous type of pad that is firm and flexible, somewhat like the cartilage in your knees. It is biconcave, or shaped like a donut with a depression in the middle but no hole. It fits somewhat like a loose baseball cap on top of the mandibular condyle (see Figure 2.4 on the next page). The disk is held in place not only by its shape but by bands of tissue that limit its movement. There is an anterior band in front and a posterior band in back. The disk sits between the mandible and temporal bones. Although the articular disk is similar to the cartilage separating the bones in your knees, it is much more active and dynamic. Unlike your knees, where the cartilage stays in place, the cartilage disk in your jaw joints moves. This can be problematic when the disk goes in the wrong direction. In your jaw joint, this is referred to as a dislocated disk. It moves independently of the condyle. This independent and complex movement is unique to the jaw joint and is necessary for your jaw to perform its many functions correctly.

The articular disk of the jaw joint is a dense, fibrous pad that is sometimes referred to as a *meniscus*. Some functions of the articular

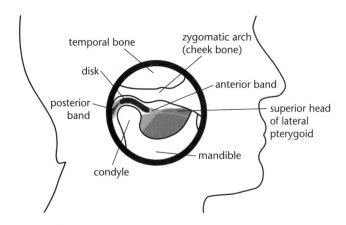

FIGURE 2.4: Articular disk, with anterior and posterior band and lateral pterygoid muscle

disk are to move like a shock absorber to help stabilize the joint and separate the bones. The disk protects the two bones of the jaw joint from rubbing together, especially during chewing and other movements. There is also a protective layer of fibrous tissue-type cartilage on the surface of the bones, where movement occurs, that protects the bones from wearing down and further reduces friction.[2] This protective layer can be more conducive to healing than that found in other joints, which is good.[3] Like the cartilage in our hips and knees, the fibrocartilage disk of the TMJ can wear out over time. Trauma and pressure can distort, damage, and tear the cartilage. Too much stress on the joints accelerates degeneration of the cartilage, as well.[4] Cartilage and joint surfaces generally wear down as we age, and cartilage can even disintegrate altogether. If this occurs, the result is bone rubbing on bone, which causes arthritis and can be painful. Protecting the disk is important and will be addressed in Chapters 3 and 9.

Synovial Joint and Joint Capsule

The TMJ is a synovial joint and produces synovial fluid that lubricates, cushions, and brings nutrients to the joint. The term *synovial* comes from the Latin word for "egg." Indeed, synovial fluid has an egg-like, stringy consistency. This fluid stays in place because a capsule surrounds the joint. The fluid is squeezed in and out like a pumping mechanism as you move the joint and is part of the reason gentle movement is healthy for the joint.

Normal movement of the TMJ creates a metabolic pump that "drives a small amount of synovial fluid in and out of the articular tissues" and brings nutrients and good stuff to the joint.[5] This fluid also lubricates the joint so there isn't as much friction. In a nutshell, this means healthy movement and the exchange of synovial fluid is good and vital for the joint to be healthy. However, sustained pressure, or joint compression, squeezes fluid out of the disk and doesn't allow it back in until the pressure releases. This sustained pressure is common in people who clench their teeth, and it can be unhealthy and hurtful. It can cause the disk to become deformed, attached to the condyle, and can narrow the disk space. If the disk is adhered or stuck, surgery is sometimes performed to release the adhesions. A displaced disk can increase tension on the joint capsule and synovial membrane. It can adversely affect the amount of fluid surrounding the joint and possibly lead to degenerative changes.

The joint capsule is a fibrous membrane and, like a balloon, it surrounds the joint and attaches the mandibular condyle to the temporal bone. Inside the balloon is the disk in the middle, synovial fluid, ligaments, and connective tissue. The balloonlike joint capsule can sometimes become irritated or inflamed, causing *capsulitis*, which literally means "inflammation of the capsule." Capsulitis can be painful and limit your ability to move your mouth.

Ligaments and the Anterior and Posterior Band

Your lower jaw, or mandible, is a loose bone that depends on a lot of structures to hold it in place. Ligaments and connective tissue are some of the structures that help hold together and stabilize the joint by limiting and restricting movement of the disk and bones. The disk is anchored in front by the anterior band and attaches to the joint capsule near the superior head of the lateral pterygoid (refer to Figure 2.4).[6] A spasm or tightness in the lateral pterygoid can adversely pull on the disk. The disk is stabilized in the back by the posterior band that combines with other vascular tissue to attach the back of the disk to the bone. The posterior band is important in limiting

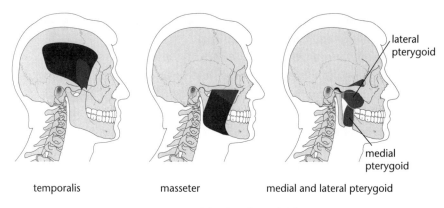

temporalis   masseter   medial and lateral pterygoid

FIGURE 2.5: Muscles of mastication

motion of the disk forward at the end of opening. If it is damaged, the disk can move too far forward and even cause your jaw to lock. Trauma such as a whiplash injury or prolonged or forceful opening of your mouth are common culprits.[7]

Some people are born with loose joints, ligaments, and tissues throughout their body, including their jaw. This is a common problem in people with TMJ disorders and is referred to as joint hypermobility, or ligamentous laxity. It is important to understand that ligaments are not elastic. If they are pulled forcibly, they don't bounce back to their original shape and size. If they are repeatedly strained and abused, they can tear and lengthen, which adversely affects the stability and function of the joint. We will talk in more detail about the disk, ligaments, connective tissue, and hypermobility in Step 7, which is found in Chapter 9.

Muscles

Your jaw muscles enable you to do many things, including chew, swallow, open and close your jaw, and move your jaw from side to side and forward and backward. Some of the primary muscles of mastication are the masseter, temporalis, medial pterygoid, and lateral pterygoid (see Figure 2.5). Muscle pain and dysfunction are the most common symptoms of TMJ disorders. We will discuss these muscles and several other supporting and stabilizing head, neck, and jaw muscles in detail in Chapter 8.

Nerves

The trigeminal nerve provides control and stimulus to important muscles that allow you to move your jaw to bite, chew, and swallow. It is the large Vth (fifth) cranial nerve and is also responsible for sensation in the face. The main nerve trunk enters the face just below the ear and near the TMJ, and then branches into three main trunks.

Trigeminal neuralgia, also known as tic douloureux, is an irritation of the trigeminal nerve and can cause episodes of mild to intense pain in the eyes, lips, nose, scalp, forehead, and jaw.[8] Occipital neuralgia is an irritation or entrapment of the occipital nerves at the base of the skull, or occiput, and is common after whiplash-type injuries. Irritation of the area due to chronic forward head posture, as is common with slouch-a-holics, or people with bifocals who repeatedly look up and down, can also irritate these nerves. Symptoms can include neck pain, headaches, dizziness, and even blurred vision. Ice, when applied to the base of the skull, often brings relief, as discussed in Chapter 10.[9]

I will also refer to the autonomic nervous system, which involves the fight-or-flight stress response, and the central nervous system, which consists of your brain, spinal cord, and your body's network of nerves. There is growing research that indicates that many people suffering from TMJ disorders and related disorders have a central nervous system that is "stuck in high gear," which can make them hypersensitive. I will use Dr Yunus's term of central sensitivity syndrome (CSS) when I refer to this phenomena.[10]

PoTSB TLC

You are now ready to start the 10 steps for establishing important healthy habits. Throughout the steps, you will see the acronym PoTSB TLC. Each letter represents a healthy habit that will help you keep your jaw in its optimal position. The acronym is arranged in an order that is easy to remember but not necessarily in order of importance. Saying the acronym will help you remember to check each of these subconscious activities that may need to be changed. PoTSB TLC is a modification of what well-known TMJ expert Steven L. Kraus calls

TTBS awareness exercises.[11] Good posture is vital to achieve these healthy habits so I have added a "Po" for posture, an "L" for lips together, and a "C" for calm and relax the muscles and mind, and rearranged the order of the steps for clarity. I will discuss each habit and exercise with you in detail in Chapters 4 through 7. These habits are essential to help you to relax and improve the health of your head, neck, and jaw. When you are not talking, chewing, or swallowing, your jaw should be at rest. Having hurtful habits can make it impossible for your jaw to rest at all, even when you are sleeping (see "Put Perfect Posture into Practice: How to Sleep" in Chapter 4).

> **Po** = Posture (Step 2)
> **T** = Tongue on the roof (Step 4)
> **S** = Swallow correctly (Step 4)
> **B** = Breathe well (Step 5)
> **TLC** = Teeth apart, Lips together, and Calm your muscles and mind (Steps 3 and 9)

Summary

Your jaw joints, or TMJs, are among the most complex joint structures in your body, and all the working parts need to function properly for long-term success. Some of these important anatomical parts include the mandible and temporal bones, the disk, joint capsule, synovial fluid, ligaments, muscles, nerves, and other associated connective tissues. Since many of these terms and structures may be new to you, feel free to refer back to Chapter 2 as needed. With a basic understanding of these components and how they work together, you are ready to dive in and examine your current behaviors to see how new healthy habits can have a positive impact on your head, neck, and jaw.

3

Step 1: Stop the Overuse and Abuse of Your Jaw

Think of the wear and tear on your jaw joints like the wear and tear on the brakes in your car. Brakes are made to stop your car and can last for years before needing to be replaced. However, if you drive with your foot on the gas and on the brake at the same time, or tap your brakes repeatedly when you are driving, your brakes will wear out more quickly. If you have hurtful habits like clenching or grinding your teeth or have a habit of chewing gum or ice for hours every day, it is somewhat like driving with your foot on the brake or repeatedly tapping the brakes, because the activity subjects the jaw joints and teeth to unnecessary wear and tear. We want to enjoy chewing, swallowing, and talking into our golden years, but unfortunately we can't just swap out our joints for new ones every thirty thousand miles. Luckily, our joints are a bit different from car brakes because they have some ability to repair and remodel—but *some* is the operative word.

When Your Joints Break Down

We all recognize that as we age, our hip and knee joints can wear down. The same holds true for our jaw joints. They are subject to wear and damage if used incorrectly. We cannot expect to hurtfully abuse them without consequence. We will touch on some hurtful habits and activities in this chapter, but many of these will be explained in greater detail in the following chapters.

You may unknowingly have hurtful habits that abuse and overuse your head, neck, and jaws and that can accelerate the wear and tear on your joints. Over time, this extra stress can lead to degenerative arthritic types of change. Your teeth can take a beating, as well. This situation is especially challenging because we are typically unaware of these habits. Health-care professionals often call these potentially hurtful oral habits *parafunctional activities*, and the following are some good examples: grinding your teeth, biting your nails, swallowing incorrectly, mouth breathing, and sucking on fingers, thumbs, and pacifiers. Most adults don't suck their thumbs, but I have worked with many who bite their lips or cheek, or chew the tags off their clothes instead.

The jaw can produce a tremendous amount of force. Just ask any dentist or hygienist who has had his or her fingers munched in somebody's mouth! So how much pressure are we talking about? Some estimates are that an adult male can generate a maximum bite load of up to 266 pounds.[1] That is the weight of some refrigerators. It shouldn't be a surprise then that clenching, grinding, and abusing your jaw joints can cause damage. Of course, having a strong bite can be useful when, for example, you want to chew a tough piece of meat grilled by your mother-in-law.

TMJ disorders are much like heart disease in that they involve a complex combination of genetic, physical, and emotional factors. The combination is different for each person. This is why I have such a passion for educating my patients to learn what they can and apply it to their own situations. You are the only one who lives with yourself twenty-four hours a day, seven days a week. You know your past and yourself better than anyone else does. As you empower yourself with the best information possible, you become the best person to decide what changes can and should be made and how to proceed.

Joint Pain

Regardless of its cause, you may have felt considerable pain associated with your TMJ disorder. Nevertheless, it is important to keep in mind that not everyone experiences the symptoms of a damaged jaw the same way. As is the case with most other joints, some people can feel horrible pain even without exhibiting any detectable degenerative joint changes. The opposite is true, as well. Other people can have dramatic degenerative changes in their joints and yet have no noticeable pain or symptoms. Thus, pain is not the only indicator of degenerative changes to the bone, although frequently the two go together.

Too many patients are inappropriately told that their pain is "all in their head," particularly when the bony surfaces of their TMJ and neck appear to be healthy. Yet there are many soft tissue structures undetectable on X rays that can be causing their pain, like muscles, nerves, ligaments, the joint capsule, and other connective tissues.

Joint Injuries

Injuries, even little ones, can play a significant role in accelerating the breakdown of joints. Many young people who already have serious deterioration and bone loss in their TMJs report being injured as a child. Maybe they fell off the counter and needed stitches in their chin. These injuries can put a chink in the armor, which in this case is the outer layer of bone, that can accelerate the deterioration and breakdown of important joint structures.[2]

Although children seldom exhibit symptoms early on as a result of injuries to the jaw, they tend to start being symptomatic in adolescence. For example, a piano teacher and mother of five said, "At age five, I fell off the slide and hit my jaw. In high school, my jaw would lock and catch. By age thirty, my jaw was locked shut and I had horrible headaches and neck pain. It took six months of effort before I could bite into a sandwich. I spent over $16,000 and had sixteen crowns and braces." Her advice to others is to "take the class" (she attended The Jaw School at Canyon Rim Physical Therapy) and do what your physical therapists and specialists say. This book is your class and will provide you with similar instruction for healthy habits.

Let's break down injuries into the common big and little ones, listing specific types of injuries that contribute to TMJ disorders. This will help you assess what you can and cannot change and what hurtful habits to focus on first.

Big Injuries

According to the American Academy of Orofacial Pain (AAOP), direct trauma has been scientifically associated with the onset of TMJ symptoms.[3] The following is a list of injuries that can have an impact on your head, neck, and jaw. In the medical world, big injuries are referred to as macrotrauma and little injuries as mictrotrauma. I have indicated in parentheses the chapter locations of the step(s) in this book where you can find help for some of these injuries.

- direct trauma or blows to the jaw (Chapter 3)
- compression of the jaw, including clenching teeth and stomach and side sleeping (Chapters 3 to 5)
- sudden overstretching of the jaw, including whiplash injuries and vomiting (Chapters 8 to 10)
- prolonged opening, as during a long dental procedure or anesthesia (Chapter 9)
- lengthy or forceful dental procedures (Chapter 9)
- joint and disk dysfunction (Chapter 9)
- pathology or disease (degenerative diseases, congenital defects) (Chapters 2 and 9)
- ligaments that are loose or damaged, making the joint less stable (Chapters 2 and 9)

Little Injuries

These activities and conditions can lead to little injuries that can add up quickly and have an effect equal to that of a big injury:

- poor posture, asymmetry, body mechanics, and neck problems (Chapters 4 and 10)
- dental issues, including missing teeth, ill-fitting crowns, fillings, or dentures (Chapter 5)
- muscular tension, teeth clenching, and grinding (Chapters 5 and 8)
- stress, anxiety, and emotional distress (Chapter 11)
- hurtful oral habits, poor tongue position and swallowing techniques (Chapters 5 to 6)

- breathing through mouth and chest (Chapter 7)
- history of hurtful oral habits like thumb sucking and pacifier use (Chapters 5 and 6)
- overopening, like that caused by a big yawn (Chapter 9)
- hurtful foods and habits (Chapter 3)
- overuse and abuse, including parafunctional activities (Chapters 3, 5, and 8)
- cervical traction that puts pressure on the jaw, including chin straps (Chapters 3 and 10)
- sleep disorders, disruption, or deficiency (Chapter 4)
- chronic infections and serious illness (Chapter 9)
- gender, genetics, your anatomy (Introduction, Chapters 2 and 9)

What You Can Do to Slow Down Wear and Tear

You cannot change your past injuries or genetic makeup, but you can improve your future. In this section, we look at some ways to counteract the subconscious hurtful habits that are within your control and that can strain and wear down your jaw joints. The first step is recognizing you are doing something hurtful. If you never learned that you weren't supposed to push the gas pedal and brake at the same time, you will have to keep replacing brake pads and could be more likely to have an accident. If you treat the symptoms of your TMJ disorder and never address or eliminate the causes or contributing factors, you may be doomed to an endless cycle of recovery and relapse.

Avoid Exerting Too Much Pressure

Avoid putting extra pressure on your jaw and neck. Some ways to do this are as follows:

- Remember TLC: Keep your Teeth apart and Lips together at rest, with Calm muscles (Step 3):
  - Do not brace, clench, or grind your teeth.
  - Your teeth should only touch momentarily when you swallow.
  - Swallowing incorrectly can strain your neck and jaw (Step 4).

- Don't keep objects between your teeth:
  - You shouldn't be smoking anyway, but cigarettes, cigars, and pipes can do additional damage to your jaw.
  - Wind instruments, whistles (common for lifeguards, coaches, and referees), and snorkels strain your jaw.
  - Avoid biting on pencils, toothpicks, your cheek, or hair.
  - For children, this may include sucking thumbs, pacifiers, bottle nipples, and biting on sippee cups.

- Avoid excessive biting, chewing, and licking:
  - Stop biting your nails, cheek, chewing gum, candy suckers, or tobacco.
  - Even licking your lips repeatedly can stress your joint.

- Avoid external pressure on the jaw:
  - Stop sleeping on your stomach and don't let your hands press on your jaw at night.
  - Use a headset or speakerphone instead of holding the phone between your ear and shoulder.
  - Stop resting your head by putting your hand under your chin.
  - Be careful using any type of chin strap.

Beware of Overuse and Fatigue

Overuse and fatigue can increase your pain and irritate your jaw. Some of the major forms of overuse to be avoided include the following:

- Poor posture.

- Incorrect jaw position.

- If you are a musician who stresses or strains your jaw (e.g., playing string, brass, or wind instruments), take frequent breaks, spread out your practice time, and pace yourself. Learn the best postures and positions in which to practice and perform. A specially trained physical therapist can use his or her knowledge of body mechanics, posture, and tools like biofeedback to help you achieve the best positions for you.

- Singing can fatigue the jaw, so pace yourself, take breaks, and beware of overopening.

- Avoid excessive talking; if you are a teacher, telemarketer, or in a profession where you must speak for hours, take breaks, incorporate the relaxation exercises you find helpful as you work through this book, and use the first-aid techniques that work best for you, as discussed in Step 8.
- Avoid excessive vomiting. If you get sick when you are pregnant, you may need to explain your jaw problem to your obstetrician and get medication to decrease your nausea and vomiting. If you are bulimic, please get some help. You are worth it!

Be Careful When Playing Sports
Sports present a special challenge for protecting the jaw. Try to protect yourself from injuries to the jaw whenever possible. As a parent, keep this in mind when you sign your child up for any type of contact sport. You can't always stop yourself or people you love from falling, and of course, you want your children to be active and have fun, but keep the following in mind:

- Beware of contact sports such as boxing, football, karate, and hockey.
- If you (or your child) must play, wear a mouth guard, use appropriate protective gear, and be cautious.

Eat and Plan Menus with Your Mouth in Mind
Your mouth is the gateway for food and you must eat to stay alive. However, some people with head, neck, and jaw problems find it too painful to eat solid food at all and resort to a liquid or soft-food diet. That stage doesn't usually last very long. A good diet is critical to health, but if you have serious jaw problems, you need to pay attention to *how* and *what* you eat to avoid overusing and abusing your TMJ.

If you have jaw problems or want to avoid extra stress and strain on your jaw joints, you should avoid the following foods:

- anything chewy, painful, or tiring
- chewing gum and ice
- hard and chewy candy

- sinewy meat, like steaks (fish and chicken are okay)
- crunchy raw vegetables (raw carrots, corn on the cob, even lettuce)
- chewy bagels and hard or chewy breads
- crunchy foods, such as nuts, tortilla chips, or peanut brittle
- caffeine, which can increase muscle tension and disturb your sleep
- mixed consistency foods, such as ice cream with nuts or yogurt with granola. Your jaw isn't always prepared for those surprise "crunchies," which can stress your muscles and jaw joints.

According to Professors Mariano Rocabado and Z. Annette Iglarsh, international experts in the field of TMJ disorders, "A soft diet and conservative joint management will add functional painless years to the life of the joint. Because people are living longer, joint conservation is essential to a healthier life."[4] Depending on the severity of your situation, you might need to be on a soft or liquid diet for a time. Even if you have no dietary restrictions, if you have chewy bagels for breakfast, a sandwich you have to stretch to get your teeth into for lunch, and a steak with raw vegetables for dinner, you might be in for a painful, sleepless night. Often, you can simply modify what and how you eat to make it easier on your joints, so try the following tips:

- Chew your food with both sides of your back teeth at the same time to ease the strain on your jaw joints and muscles.
- Cut food into small pieces, peel apples and other skinned food.
- Cook fruits and vegetables or mix raw fruits and vegetables into smoothies.
- Toast your bagels and/or dip your chewy breads into something moist.
- Drinking water is important, but rocking your head back repeatedly to drink can irritate your neck. Try using a straw unless sucking a straw irritates your jaw.

A healthy diet can go a long way toward helping your body recover more quickly from an injury and can help prevent degeneration of your joints. So eat wisely! Eat a good, balanced diet consisting of foods such as cooked whole grains, beans, vegetables, eggs, fish, cheese, ground meats, and fruit. Refer to the U.S. Dietary Guidelines at http://www.health.gov/DietaryGuidelines to help you make healthy food choices.[5] Talk to your doctor about appropriate supplements. Patients with damage to their jaw joints may want to discuss taking glucosamine chondroitin. Nutritional inadequacies are essential to address in the management of muscle pain. Travell and Simons point out that of particular concern are the vitamins B-1, B-6, B-12, folic acid, and vitamin C, and the elements calcium, iron, and potassium.[6] Discuss these supplements with your doctor. You can get general information from the National Institutes of Health Office of Dietary Supplements at http://ods.od.nih.gov.

Summary

Now that your eyes have been opened up to the ways you unwittingly add wear and tear on your jaw joints, it is time to make your own checklist for change so you can start replacing any hurtful habits with healthy ones.

1. Identify any ways you put extra stress and strain on your jaw joints. Include major and minor stressors, as even the small stressors add up.

2. Make a plan to eliminate or decrease the hurtful habits that can be wearing down your jaw joints.

3. Plan a two-week menu of healthy, nonirritating foods and snacks you enjoy. Peel, cut, cook, and dip your foods as needed to help your jaw in the chewing process. Evaluate your nutritional needs with your doctor.

4. Make yourself a personalized checklist for change. Use Table 3.1 on the next page as a guide.

Table 3.1: Checklist for Change: Eliminating Abuse and Overuse

HURTFUL HABIT	HEALTHY HABIT	CHECKLIST FOR CHANGE
I hold the phone to my ear when I talk.	Instead, I will use a headset or speakerphone when I talk on the phone or will send a text message.	I will buy a headset for my cell and home phone and learn how to use my speakerphones and text message.
I excessively chew gum, ice, and pencils.	I will decrease the stress to my jaw joints by only chewing what is necessary.	I will not buy or chew gum and will not put ice in my drinks. I will freshen my breath with a small, quickly dissolving mint. I will wrap my pencils in felt to discourage me from chewing on them.
I play the violin for one to two hours at a time.	I will minimize the strain that musical instruments can pose to my jaws and neck.	I will break up my practice times into smaller blocks. I will improve the postures and positions I am in to minimize strains while playing and may seek the help of a specialist.

4

Step 2: The Power of Posture
Learn How to Stand, Sit, and Sleep

Are you a slouch-a-holic? Perhaps your mother told you to stand up straight. And maybe you didn't listen, and over the years you developed into a slouch-a-holic, someone who habitually slouches forward. Your mother was right, but did she tell you exactly how to correct your posture? Did she tell you the best positions in which to stand, sit, and sleep? After reading this chapter, which focuses on the **Po** in PoTSB TLC, or posture, you will know the answers and should be able to give her a tip or two.

Why You Want Good Posture

Let me begin by telling you about a patient I had early in my career who changed the way I think. Working with him helped me realize the power and importance of good posture and positioning.

William: Changing His Posture Was the Key

As a young physical therapist, I was assigned William, a middle-aged man diagnosed with terminal cancer that had spread throughout his body, including his spine. He had difficulty sleeping, shaving, and getting around. At first, I wasn't exactly sure what I could do for him. I started by focusing on his postures and positions. He was an author and incredibly bright and motivated. We got to work by addressing his sleeping posture and by me teaching him the simple concepts I will teach you later in this chapter. It wasn't long before he was sleeping soundly for most of the night. Then we found the best posture and position for him to use when he shaved his face. And finally, we got him exercising. Before I discharged him, he was able to walk an hour or more a day with his lovely wife, and he was sleeping through the night and able to shave without any difficulties. Many would have written off this man, thinking there was nothing that could be done for him. Yet, after a few simple visits and a willingness to make changes, he was able to truly live and more fully enjoy the rest of the life that he had. It was a sobering lesson I have never forgotten.

So what do posture and positioning have to do with your head, neck, and jaw? The answer is everything! Posture is the foundation for movement and function. Proper posture and balancing of your head is essential in achieving the most relaxed head, neck, and jaw positions and the foundation for the healthy habits you want to form.

Your Heavy Head

When people think about posture, they often think about the position of their head. Do you know how heavy your head is? The average head weighs approximately 10 to 12 pounds.[1] In other words, your head is heavier than a gallon of milk. That gallon of milk (your head) is balanced carefully on a stick (your spine), with a bunch of bands (muscles, tissue, and ligaments) to help hold it in place. Now imagine if that gallon of milk is not balanced, but is tipping forward. Instead of the 12-pound weight being supported vertically throughout your system, your neck must struggle to support up to 36 pounds of pressure (see Figure 4.1).[2] This situation will cause wear and tear on the spine as well as on the muscles and supporting structures that must work all day to support this extra load that is three times heavier than it needs to be if it were balanced. Balance will be an important concept as we talk about posture and positions.

One of the reasons so many of us have sore necks is that we consistently use some form of a forward head posture. Researchers recently confirmed that a forward head posture pushes the mandibular condyle backward.[3] Professors Mariano Rocabado and Z. Annette

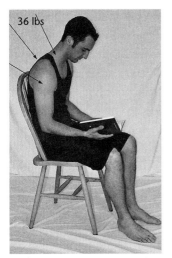
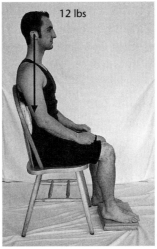
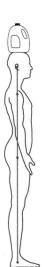

36 lbs

12 lbs

FIGURE 4.1: Balanced posture, standing and sitting

Iglarsh reported a 70 percent correlation between having a forward head posture and a lower jaw that is pushed back, or retruded.[4] This condition is called *mandibular,* or *condylar, retrusion,* and according to Dr. Robert Talley, it can lead to the following TMJ-related problems:[5]

- pinches the pad behind the disk (retrodiscal pad)
- damages TMJ metabolism
- reduces the TMJ blood supply
- stretches out the ligaments
- stretches and strains the lateral pterygoid muscle and can cause it to go into spasm
- wears away the posterior disk band

The previous list illustrates how poor posture can adversely impact the jaw joints. However, there are even more unfortunate consequences for slouch-a-holics.

The Price of Bad Posture

According to the American Physical Therapy Association's guidelines on posture, good posture can help "your body function at top

speed. It promotes movement efficiency and endurance and con-
tributes to an overall feeling of well-being...poise, confidence, and
dignity."[6] Therefore, lousy posture would tend to have the opposite
effect: slowing you down, decreasing efficiency and endurance, and
perhaps even contributing to depression and poor self-esteem. They
go on to say that poor posture can strain your muscles, joints, and
ligaments, and eventually lead to fatigue and pain. In addition, when
slouch-a-holics hang their heads forward, it can throw their systems
off balance and out of whack, including their neck and jaw. They may
clench their jaws, thrust their tongues, and swallow incorrectly as
a result.[7] This can cause headaches and neck and jaw pain, and can
contribute to incorrect breathing and swallowing (see Chapter 6
on swallowing and Chapter 7 on breathing). It speeds up the wear
and tear on your spine and joints, putting you in the fast lane to pain
or dysfunction. Your muscles work overtime as well, making them
tense, tight, and sore. In a study by Japanese researchers, patients
who received postural training for daily life activities had less muscle
pain and were able to open their mouths wider than those who had
not received postural training.[8]

I have used the terms *neutral* and *balanced* throughout this book.
These terms are often used when talking about joints and muscles
and in general means that the joints or muscles are in their mid-
range, or balanced, position. This is typically a more relaxed and
healthier position. I often tell my patients to think of their muscles
as if they were pieces of paper. When they are in a neutral position, it
is like their muscles are a flat, relaxed piece of paper, but when they
are shortened or compressed for long periods, it is like crumpling the
paper. While the muscles and ligaments of our bodies are much more
flexible than paper, it is important to move and stretch the muscles
and joints through their full, healthy range of healthy motion and to
remember that you cannot stress and strain them for prolonged periods of time without eventual consequences.

Imagine if you were to sleep all night on your stomach with
your arm overhead, your neck twisted and jaw smashed against the
bed—you would be twisting, crumpling, and crushing many of your
muscles and joints, and pulling on others the entire night. In the

morning, though, you would somehow expect them to be flat and balanced, and to feel good. It seems that the majority of my patients with the worst damage to their jaw joints sleep on their stomach or on their sides with their hand pushing on their jaw all night. I even had a patient herniate a disc in her neck after sleeping on her stomach with her neck twisted.

The same holds true for prolonged work positions or daily postures. You must learn where neutral is and how to achieve balance in your postures and then apply that knowledge to your various activities.

Our body parts are all connected. When one part of the body is out of balance, it adversely affects the other parts. These parts then have to adjust to accommodate. The neck, back, and shoulder muscles that support the head can also refer pain to other structures, such as your face, ears, eyes, and head. Other odd symptoms sometimes associated with poor posture include dizziness, ringing in your ears, nausea, blurred vision, intestinal distress, and sleep apnea. Additional problems include disk dysfunction and degenerative arthritis.[9]

How to Assess Your Posture

Now that you know a bit more about the importance of good posture to your health, let's try to get a realistic picture of your true posture right now. Assessing your own posture can help you know if you need professional help, in addition to improving your awareness and balance with some "do-it-yourself" techniques.

In order to see the important body landmarks, it is best to assess your posture while in your underwear (bra and panties for ladies, briefs for gentlemen), without shoes or socks, and while standing on a hard, level floor. To do all the assessments, you will need a full-length mirror and a partner, or a camera with a self-timer. To get a realistic picture, it is also important that you relax and stand the way you normally stand instead of how you think you should be standing.

You will want to assess your posture from all angles: from the front, back, and side view positions. You can take a picture of yourself in the mirror from each angle or get your friend to take a picture. Photos must capture your full body from head to toe and should be set up as level as possible. As I look at patients, I often make a rough sketch that gives me a general idea of their posture. If you do not have a camera, a friend may be able to make observations or draw rough sketches, or you can try looking at the same landmarks in a mirror. After you have looked yourself over once, get a pen and paper and write down your findings as you reassess yourself. You may want to recheck yourself periodically over a week or two in order to get a more accurate assessment.

Back- or Front-View Assessment

The back view is how I prefer to start assessing posture, because I can see the spine and shoulder blades, but it is much more difficult for someone at home alone to do so. I look at many of the same landmarks as for the front view, but with the back view, I can also feel for and assess curves or abnormalities in the person's spine and the position of the shoulder blades. If you have a friend to help you, he or she can assess you from the back and then take a photo or draw a sketch. Otherwise, you can assess yourself by standing in front of a full-length mirror on a firm level surface in your underwear. We will work our way from head to toes (see Figure 4.2):

1. Are you smiling? You should smile at yourself because you are doing yourself a service by reading and applying the principles in this book. Hooray for you!

2. Is your head tilted to one side or the other? If so, toward which side does your head tilt?

3. Is one shoulder higher than the other? If so, which one is higher?

4. Is one arm next to or closer to your body than the other arm? If so, which one?

5. Is one pelvis or "hip bone" higher than the other?

6. Looking at the back, is one shoulder blade higher than the other or are they level?

7. Looking at the back, is the spine straight, or does it curve?

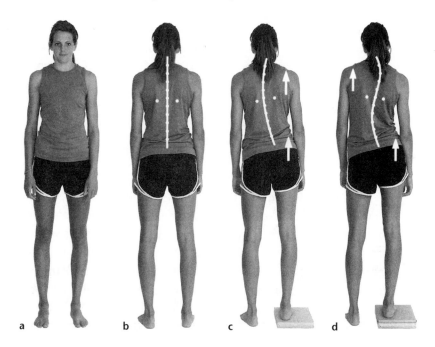

FIGURE 4.2: Front and back views of posture: (a) front view, balanced; (b) back view, balanced; (c) back view, high right hip and right shoulder with compensatory spinal curve; and (d) back view, high right hip and left shoulder with compensatory spinal curve

Seeking Professional Help for Postural Problems

It is good for your body and its postures to be balanced. If you answered yes to any of the self-assessment questions, you may want to see a qualified health-care provider trained in evaluating posture to obtain further assessment. You can bring your pictures, findings, and this information to your appointment so the provider can evaluate you more carefully. The following are some of the things he or she can check for.

Leg-Length Discrepancy

A large discrepancy in leg length can have a profound effect on your posture, your jaw, and all the joints as you move up the body. It may be easier to imagine it this way; Think of your pelvis as the tabletop and your legs as the legs of the table. Then imagine the bones in your spine as wooden blocks, with disks or jelly donuts between each segment in a tall pillar in the center of the table. At the very top of this pillar is a 10-pound medicine ball representing your head. Now imagine that the legs on the left side of the table are shorter. This would tip the table to the left, and the ball on top representing your head would probably fall. Luckily, we have other structures to help provide stabilization, but having to use these structures to keep the head balanced would still be a continuous strain on the system.

I have tried to simulate the effects of a leg-length difference in Figures 4.2c and 4.2d on the previous page. I have placed one and then two books under the model's right leg in these pictures so you can see how the spine, shoulders, and head compensate to balance the head so you don't have to look at the world with your head tipped at an angle. It is interesting to note that with one book under the right leg the model's same-side shoulder is elevated (see Figure 4.2c), but with two books under the right leg the model compensates by elevating the opposite shoulder (see Figure 4.2d).

Some medical professionals estimate that 60 to 90 percent of the general population have one leg somewhat longer than the other.[10] Don't think you are malformed if you have a leg-length difference. Many parts of our bodies are a bit asymmetrical: our face, arms, and legs. When I reach my arms out in front of me, it is very clear my right arm is longer. But I don't walk on my arms, so it doesn't have the same impact a leg-length difference would have. It is only necessary to correct an asymmetry if it is causing a problem.

Travell and Simons say the only way to precisely measure leg length is with a standing X ray.[11] You can almost always avoid unnecessary radiation by having a trained professional evaluate you in several positions. It is important to differentiate between a true leg-length difference and tight muscles or an imbalance in the pelvis that can create what appears to be a difference in the length of your legs but is not. A trained clinician can assess this in several ways. One way is for you to sit on a flat surface with your legs straight out and then again lying down. If there is any change in leg length from the sitting position to the lying-down position, more investigation is needed.

If a true leg-length difference is found, I usually determine how much correction is needed, based on the person's condition and their age. I tend to correct younger people in full, whereas with older people who have accommodated to the differences, we tend to correct less because they have tolerated this condition longer and may not tolerate correction as easily as would younger people. I usually make a correction by putting a heel lift or pad inside of the shoe. Heel lifts bigger than ⅜ inch are rarely needed. Large corrections may require special shoes.

Sam: One Leg Too Short

Sam, a teenage boy, came to me for treatment, complaining of TMJ pain just on one side. Upon examination, we found one of his legs was significantly longer than the other. We performed several tests to be sure it was a true leg-length discrepancy. We decided to try an experiment. Initially, we treated him with only a heel lift, which he wore inside his shoe to decrease the leg-length discrepancy and help level his posture. We were a bit surprised when his jaw felt 50 percent improved by the time of his next visit. Who would have thought that treating him at the foot could have improved his jaw so significantly? But then again, our bodies are one long kinetic chain connecting us from head to toe.

Pelvic Asymmetry

A leg-length difference isn't the only structural problem that can affect your posture. While it is much less common, one side of your pelvis can be smaller than the other side. Often referred to as a hemi-pelvis, this could require a lift under one buttock to level your posture in sitting, as well as a heel lift to help you stand on the shorter side.

Your spine sits on your pelvis, so any shift or asymmetry of the pelvis can affect the position of the spine and shoulders and make it appear that you have a leg-length difference when you really do not.[12] Remember to look for causes. A fall or a poor sleeping position every night can adversely affect the position of the pelvis. If you have an unstable pelvis, something as simple as merely sitting down when you put on your pants and shoes can help keep this important area stable, especially if you have a weak core and abdominals. A physical therapist trained in orthopedics can assess your pelvis and sacrum and help realign them using gentle stretches, exercises, and manual or muscle energy techniques, and then help you strengthen and balance your core and the structures that surround the pelvis to regain stability. Many of those suffering from TMJ-related disorders have loose joints, as in the following example.

Pillow-Pinching Penny

Penny had daily headaches and loose ligaments. In fact, her joints were so loose, you could hear her pelvis *clunk* when she walked. Postural evaluation showed a leg-length discrepancy. However, her leg length changed when she shifted from a long sitting position, where she sat with her legs straight in front of her, to a supine position on her back, with her pelvis rotated. I wanted to start as gently as possible, so I tried a simple pillow pinch, or squeeze. While lying on her back, Penny would squeeze a folded pillow gently between her knees three or four times, using about 50 percent of her maximum force capability. This simple exercise was enough to help rebalance Penny's pelvis, and her leg-length discrepancy disappeared. Penny tried this exercise every night before going to bed and reported that when she would pinch the pillow at night, she would not have a headache the next day.

Scoliosis Can Throw a Curve in Your Posture

Scoliosis is a lateral, or side-to-side, curve of the spine and it can throw off your posture and thus the balance of your head, neck, and jaw. However, not all types of scoliosis are caused by a structural abnormality in the spine. If you have a leg-length discrepancy or hemipelvis, your spine sits on an uneven base, or table, which forces your spine to curve to compensate and balance your head, creating a functional scoliosis as seen in Figures 4.2c and 4.2d on page 35. A functional scoliosis is usually easily resolved when the discrepancy is resolved, like with a heel lift. The muscles and soft tissues may have accommodated as well and a physical therapist can prescribe exercises and stretches to restore the balance and stability of your spine.

You can also have a combination of both a functional and structural scoliosis. If you think you have scoliosis, be sure to be evaluated by a specialist to determine what, if any, treatment is needed.

Side-View Measurement

You will need to see your ear, shoulder, hip, knee, and ankle. If you have long hair, you may want to pull your hair behind your ear. Stand sideways on a firm, level surface facing the edge of a wall or doorway. If your walls are straight, this edge will serve as a type of plumb line, or vertical guide, as you look at your picture. Have your friend (or camera on self-timer) take a couple of pictures of you from the side. Make sure the camera is level and includes the bottom of your feet all the way up to the top of your head. If you don't have a camera, your friend can make a sketch. Do not read the next paragraph until you have taken your picture or you may be tempted to cheat by standing how you are supposed to stand instead of how you really do.

After you have taken your side-view picture, print the picture and then use a pen to put dots on your anklebone, knee, hip, shoulder, and ear. (You can place dots on yourself before you take pictures as well—tattoos are not necessary.) Using a ruler or straightedge, draw a line from one dot to another as illustrated in Figure 4.3a on the next page. Your eventual goal is to be able to create a straight line as you connect the dots from just in front of your anklebone, up to the middle of your knee, through your hip (greater trochanter), shoulder, and lobe of your ear.[13] This does not mean your spine is straight. Even with these landmarks making a straight line, there should be a small curve (or *lordosis*) in the lumbar spine (or the small of your back where a belt would go), and a small curve in the back of your neck, as depicted in Figure 4.3a on the next page.[14]

How Do You Measure Up?

If your dots don't line up, you can join the ranks of the other slouch-a-holics and take the first step on the road to recovery, which is to recognize there is a problem. Even though I have taught hundreds of people the importance of good posture, I still occasionally catch myself slumping. Gravity pushes down against us all the time with a force of 9.8 meters/sec^2. It takes work to fight against gravity the

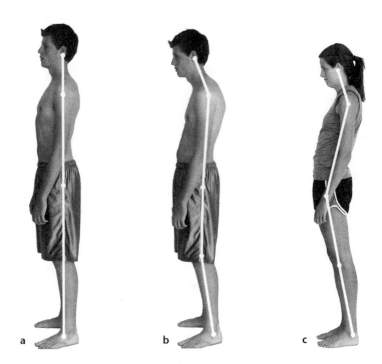

FIGURE 4.3: Side views of postures: (a) balanced posture,
(b) unbalanced posture, and (c) unbalanced posture

entire day. Nevertheless, we can fight back with reminders and a few strategically placed supports.

As is often the case, there are some exceptions to keep in mind. Some people will never be able to achieve perfect alignment. Diseases and disorders such as scoliosis and osteoporosis can prevent some people from achieving ideal posture. However, by working with your health-care professionals, you can work toward it, using whatever modifications are necessary for your situation in order to maintain your best posture possible.

Put Perfect Posture into Practice:
How to Stand

When we talk about how to find your correct or balanced posture, we start from the bottom of the body and work our way up. When you stand, posture starts with your feet.

Your Standing Posture, Foot to Head

If you completed the exercise above and took a picture of yourself from the side, you should be able to draw a line from your ankle, hip, shoulder, and ear and see three normal balanced curves in your back (see Figure 4.3a or Figure 4.1a on page 31). Let's look at the elements of your standing posture according to your body parts involved and discuss them one by one.

Feet

Start by shifting your body weight so that you feel your weight balanced over your arch or middle of your feet. Your weight should not rest on the back of your heels or front of your toes. Wear good supportive shoes and avoid high heels (including boots) that mess up your posture. If you have flat feet or loose ligaments, you might benefit from good arch supports. You can try inexpensive arch supports at your local pharmacy or talk to your physical therapist or foot specialist.

- Hide your high-heeled footwear in the attic or just toss them out.

- For those dressier shoes with no support, try to find a quality arch support that you can transfer from shoe to shoe as needed.

- Try wearing a good supportive pair of house shoes instead of going barefoot at home.

Knees

Your knees should be straight. If you stand with your knees bent, you may have tight hamstrings (see Chapter 11). You also need to make sure your knees are not hyperextended or buckled backward. If this is your typical way of standing, it may feel like your knees are slightly bent, but they are actually now in a balanced neutral position. This can be a common problem for people with TMJ disorders and hypermobile joints. If you think of yourself as "double jointed," be sure to read Chapter 9, in which we discuss joint hypermobility. You would likely benefit from strengthening the muscles around the knee and learning how to protect your joints. A physical therapist trained in orthopedics can help you.

Hips and Pelvis

Many people throw their hips forward as if they were wearing high heels (see Figure 4.3c on page 40). Others rotate their pelvis backward as if they are tucking under a tail (see Figure 4.3b on page 40). This is frequently caused by tight hamstrings or quadricep hip flexors. Stretches such as those illustrated in Chapter 11 or other stretches decided on with your provider may be an important step in attaining the flexibility required to achieve those balanced curves you need for good posture. If your muscles are tight and are adversely affecting your posture, safely stretch them each day for two weeks and then after any time you walk or exercise. Common culprits are the hamstrings, quadriceps, and calf muscles. You may add the stretches found in Chapter 11 to your routine. (Ask your physical therapist for stretches specific to your situation and also review the exercises described in Chapter 11.)

Abdominals

Don't just hang on your abs, tone and train them. Because diaphragmatic, or belly breathing, is so important, you must find that delicate balance between having taut and toned abdominals and still being able to breathe using your diaphragm, which expands your rib cage and abdominal muscles. Typically, the deep abdominals are weak and yet are important stabilizers for good posture.

Back

If you look at the picture of your back, your spine should be straight and balanced as seen in Figure 4.2b on page 35. However, in the picture of you from the side, you should have natural curves in your spine that need to be balanced for you to stand in proper alignment and to balance your head, neck, and jaw (see Figure 4.3a on page 40). The curve in the back of your neck is your cervical curve, and the curve in your lower back is your lumbar curve. Typically, you can balance your head and stand in good posture simply by elongating your spine as in the "posture quick fix" on page 46 so that your ankle, hip, shoulder, and ear are aligned (again see Figure 4.3a). However, be patient. You can't undo years of poor posture overnight. It takes time and sometimes the help of a professional.

Shoulders

Most people's shoulders become rounded from slouching or sleeping on their side. Look at yourself in the mirror while facing forward. Stand naturally. If your shoulders are back and your thumbs are facing forward, you are probably in good shape. However, if you see the back of your hand, your shoulders are probably rounded and your pectoralis muscles are probably tight. Try standing erect and then imagine a string tied to the top of your sternum or breastbone and then lift the string. Usually this helps your shoulders naturally move back into a more balanced position. Stretching your pectoralis muscles can help you achieve a balanced posture. There are multiple ways to stretch a muscle. If you have loose joints or are prone to dislocating your shoulder, you should consult your doctor or physical therapist to determine if you should include the pectoralis stretches on pages 164 and 165 (Figures 8.22 and 8.23) in your after-exercise stretching routine. Because the majority of us have a forward head posture with rounded shoulders, this in turn affects our shoulders and scapula (shoulder blades), often pulling them apart. Tight pecs and rounded shoulders can make it difficult for the middle and lower trapezius muscles to do their job and can create a weakness and postural imbalance that may need specialized exercises designed by a physical therapist. There are many variables that are beyond the scope of this book to address, but scapular stability could be an important step in achieving a balanced posture and healthy movement patterns.

Head, Eyes, and Mandible

Your head should be balanced, with your eyes pointed forward, not looking up or down. This can pose a problem if you wear bifocals or trifocals and must routinely glance up and down to switch lenses. Consider getting a separate pair of glasses for specific tasks like working on the computer or reading. A forward head posture will put tension on the muscles.[15] In proper posture, your tongue can more easily anchor/rest on the roof of your mouth, which helps relax your jaw muscles with your teeth apart. This makes you less likely to clench your teeth together.

Common Standing Posture Problems and Solutions

Let's look at some of the most common and problematic positions and activities that occur while standing. For each, I offer helpful solutions.

Standing with an uneven distribution of weight. A majority of my patients like to stand with their weight on one leg, with their hip pushed to one side as if they are holding a baby (see Figures 4.4e and f, "unbalanced"). This pose usually creates a type of functional scoliosis and strains your muscles and joints by pulling unevenly. Instead, stand with your weight on both feet. If you need to change positions, it is better to shift your weight with one foot in front of the other or evenly from side to side. This helps you stand up straight and in a balanced position (see Figures 4.4a and b, "balanced").

Standing in the same position for a long time...like during shaving or while putting on makeup. The solutions are simple: Stagger your feet and put an arm down for support. You can even open the cupboard to make room for your staggered front foot (see Figure 4.4d). Also, change positions frequently. Try to change positions every 20 to 30 minutes, or as needed. You can lean back against a wall for support or change position by putting a foot on some type of footrest or low chair and alternate as needed (see Figure 4.4b). Think through ways to apply balanced postures to all your standing activities like doing the dishes, cooking, etc.

Lifting or carrying something heavy. First, do NOT clench your teeth when doing a strenuous activity. Carrying a purse, briefcase, bag, backpack, or child will usually throw off your posture and strain your head, neck, and jaw (see Figure 4.4f). Carry as little as possible. Buy an extra set of what you need (this doesn't apply to children) and leave it at the office and in the car instead of lugging it around everywhere every day. If you have to carry something, hold the weight close to your body near your center of gravity, which is typically against your belly or the small of your back (see Figure 4.4c). Distribute the weight evenly by using fanny packs or backpacks with a hip strap or a backpack purse and use both straps. Whenever possible, use rolling

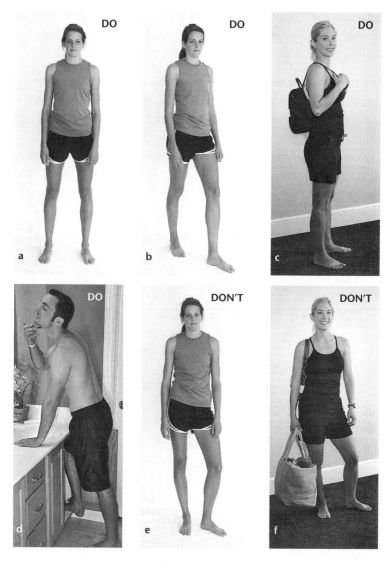

FIGURE 4.4: Standing do's "balanced" (a, b, c, d)
and don'ts "unbalanced" (e, f)

bags, strollers, and so forth to unload. Lifting or moving 10 pounds
when it is next to your center of gravity adds 10 pounds, but at arm's
length, it can seem like more than an additional 100 pounds on your
spine.[16] Yet, you do this every time you take your 10-pound purse or

briefcase and reach out to place it on the floor of the passenger's side of your car, and you strain your neck and shoulder in the process. Put it in the trunk or backseat instead.

Leaning forward toward a mirror or over the sink. When leaning forward to shave or apply makeup, or over the sink to do dishes, open the cupboard underneath and stagger your feet one in front of the other by resting one foot just inside the cupboard. Rest your hips against the edge. If leaning forward, put one arm down to support your body weight in a neutral, balanced position (see Figure 4.4d). Or better yet, buy a mirror that can be moved toward you. Avoid twisting your body haphazardly (e.g., by trying to drink directly from the faucet—keep a cup by the sink instead).

Walking. Maintain good posture while walking. Look straight ahead instead of at the floor or ceiling, which could strain your neck and jaw. People with TMJ disorders are often tense. You should feel comfortable and balanced but not stiff. Each arm should move rhythmically in conjunction with the opposite leg.

A Posture Quick Fix

Because most of us are short on time, you need a posture "quick fix," which is an easy way to balance your posture quickly. The following simple exercises and imagery usually do the trick:

- Imagine there is a string tied to the crown or back of your head and you are being lifted by that string toward the ceiling. You should feel balanced, elongated, and energized. Smiling helps, too.

- Next, lift the imaginary string attached to your sternum or breastbone. This helps rounded shoulders roll back into place. Go easy! Do not make yourself uncomfortable.

Tall Tom: Years of Back Pain Managed in Just a Few Weeks

I had a middle-aged man named Tom come for treatment, presenting with chronic back pain. For over a year, he went weekly for a manipulation that brought quick relief, but his symptoms always returned. He was tall and his posture was abysmal. His hamstrings were so tight that they rotated his pelvis backward, making it look as if his bottom was tightly tucked underneath him. This posterior pelvic tilt flattened the important curves in his spine, causing a forward head posture. He was stiff, slouched, and miserable. I taught him the basics of good posture and stressed the extreme importance of good posture, and I also gave him many of the exercises we will discuss in Chapter 11, Step 9, which were essential to helping him achieve good posture. He was a quick learner, hard worker, and otherwise healthy man. In two to three weeks, he was 70 to 80 percent improved and able to manage his progress on his own.

Put Perfect Posture into Practice: How to Sit

Because many of us spend more time sitting than standing, let's build on the healthy habits you have learned in standing and add some simple principles for sitting. You still want your landmarks (hip, ear, and shoulder) to line up. However, your feet will be in a different part of the lineup, so let's start there.

Your Sitting Posture, Foot to Head

To learn how to sit correctly, let's start in a chair. We always start at the foundation or bottom of the body. In sitting, it is literally your bottom and the surfaces you are resting on, which are your feet on the floor and your bottom on the seat. Then we will work our way up to your head.

Feet and Legs

Wherever you sit, your feet should be able to reach the floor or rest on a stable footrest in front of your knees. This is a common problem for my shorter patients. If money is tight, I recommend saving old phone books, wrapping them with tape, and using them as inexpensive footrests. Sometimes I pull out the bottom drawer of my desk to rest one foot on the drawer, alternating as needed. You can be creative and use whatever is available, whether it be magazines, books, or a properly placed backpack on the floor of an airplane, to rest your feet on. Avoid crossing your legs, as it can twist your body and create an unnatural curve in your spine that can throw your head, neck, and jaw off balance. Most of my patients have a tendency to always cross the same leg, which can make one hip tighter than the other. I prefer they don't cross their legs at all, but if they do, I recommend they be balanced and evenly stretch both sides of the body.

Bottom

First, take your wallet and keys out of your pocket. These can press on nerves and throw off your posture. Adjust your chair to the correct height for you if you have that option. Scoot your bottom all the way to the back of the chair so your sacrum and pelvis can't roll backward. If you are in a deep chair or couch, you can place a pillow behind you to shorten the distance and support your back and pelvis. If your pelvis is not supported, it has a tendency to roll backward, causing you to slump. You can also sit on the edge of a chair or stool for short periods; this tilts your pelvis forward to maintain a normal lumbar curve but can put somewhat more strain on your back. Resting some of your weight on your feet can help. Changing positions is good. Your body is made to move and it is healthier when you do. I wiggle around in my chair and stand up and stretch about every twenty minutes. The strains of work and sitting at a computer for long periods can irritate your head and neck.[17] Use these principles as a guide and find what works best for you. Later in this section I provide information on how to adjust your workstation and chair more ergonomically (see Figure 4.6 on page 54 as well).

Back

According to Dr. Alan Hedge, director of Ergonomics at Cornell University, the back of your chair should slope at an angle of 100 to 110 degrees,[18] which is 10 to 20 degrees backward from the straight-up position. If the back is too straight, it is difficult to feel relaxed, and you may slide your hips forward, which ruins your good posture.

Next, your back should feel supported. Some fancy ergonomic chairs support your lower and upper back; however, if you do not have a supportive ergonomic type of chair, the easiest thing to do is to place a back support behind the middle or small of your back. This

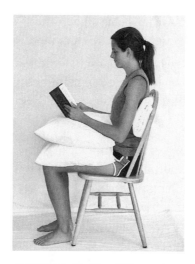

FIGURE 4.5: Healthy sitting posture

is about where a normal belt would go and will support the normal curve of your lumbar spine. You should have a support in every chair or seat you spend time in, including your computer chair, car, and couch. You can consider purchasing inflatable back supports to carry with you, because you never know when you might be sitting and need a back support.

You can purchase a variety of chairs and back supports. Make sure you choose one that is comfortable and the right size for you. It is a big plus if you can attach the support to the chair to keep it in the right place at the small of your back. This is critical because I have seen many well-meaning people with their back supports fallen to the bottom of their chair actually pushing them into worse posture than without the support.

Some inexpensive back support ideas include the following (for more back support ideas go to www.tmjhealingplan.com):

- A small folded hand towel works well (see Figure 4.5). You can attach it to your seatback with straps or Velcro.

- Inflatable water wings are inexpensive and portable if you can find the right kind. Cut them along the seam so that they open up, and apply Velcro to hold them in place. You can adjust the amount of air depending on the surface you are sitting on. Of course there are also inflatable supports for sale that are created just for this purpose and that are much more comfortable.

- You can also use what is available wherever you go. On an airplane, I use a pillow or blanket. In a waiting room, I might use a magazine as a back support. In church, I use the hymn book.

Arms

When sitting for long periods, it can help to give your neck and shoulders a break by supporting your arms with half armrests, which are just long enough to support your elbows and part of your forearm. If you have full-length armrests, they can prevent you from being able to position yourself close enough to the desk and can get in your way as you get in an out of your chair. If the armrests are too low, try to adjust them or wrap them with towels so they can adequately support the weight of your shoulder girdle, which includes your arms, shoulders, and supporting musculature. However, it is best if the armrests can move out of the way so your elbows can move freely when you are typing. If typing is your primary task, then it may be best to have no armrests at all.

While watching television, use extra pillows to relieve your neck muscles from having to support the weight of your arms and shoulders. The armrests in the car are often too far apart for my smaller patients. For long drives, some patients place a pillow next to them to rest their arms. Your shoulder girdle amounts to about 14 percent of your body weight.[19] If you weigh 120 pounds, the effort expended in supporting your shoulder girdle is like carrying 16 to 17 pounds (almost two gallons of milk) around all day. This extra weight is literally a pain in the neck. Other ways to take the load off include the following:

- When you are standing, put your hands on your hips or in your pockets.
- Wear a fanny pack instead of carrying a purse.
- Keep the things you need most within reach of your bent arms when your shoulders are relaxed and your elbows are at your sides, because reaching strains your neck. This is a common

problem when people position their computer mouse too far away or too high.

- Keep your elbows free while typing. When you are not typing or need a break, rest your elbows on the armrests.

Head and Eyes

Your head should be upright, not tilted to one side or the other. The following tips will help to keep your head properly aligned:

- Remember not to cradle the telephone between your shoulder and your ear. Instead, use a headset or speakerphone.

- Place your computer terminal directly in front of you, about arm's length away, with the top of the viewing screen just above eye level (see Figure 4.6 on page 54). Use a document holder.

- Bifocals and trifocals require you to look up and down constantly, which can irritate your neck. Consider having separate pairs of glasses, particularly when doing one activity for a long time.

- To reduce eyestrain, remember the 20/20/20 rule: Every 20 minutes look 20 feet away for 20 seconds.[20] Beware of glare, reflections, and too much or too little light. This is also a great time to take a microbreak to stretch and move as well.

Common Sitting Posture Problems and Solutions

Here are some of the most common and problematic positions and activities that occur while sitting, and some helpful solutions.

Reading and Writing

- It is common for people to read a note or newspaper at a table by bending over or slouching their whole body over to read, instead of lifting the lightweight paper up to them and staying in good posture. When possible, lift the book or paper up to you instead. You can use pillows to support the book and balance your posture as seen in Figure 4.5 on page 49.

- Slanted writing surfaces like a drafting table are ideal for keeping your head upright.

- When working at a computer, use a document holder that lifts the paper to eye level and brings it closer to the screen, which prevents you from rotating your head at an awkward angle for prolonged periods, and switch sides occasionally so you are not always looking the same direction.

Watching Television

- Adjust your television so you can watch it straight on at the right height. Turning your head at an angle for long periods can cause headaches and neck pain.

- Do not watch television while you are lying back in a recliner or in bed. Unless your television is on the ceiling, you will have to strain your head forward to see the TV. Sit up straight while watching and recline while reading or resting.

Sitting for Long Periods

Sitting for long periods can cause blood to pool in your legs. Stand up and walk around to get your circulation moving and help you think more clearly. When purchasing a new desk, consider one that allows you to alternate sitting or standing. In one clinic where I worked, we set our laptops on rolling bed trays that adjusted up and down. They were cheap and versatile.

Driving a Car

In the car, you should apply the principles above and also be aware of the following:[21]

- Your knees should be slightly lower than your hips.

- Your seat should be upright enough that your hips are close to a 90-degree angle.

- Ensure adequate lumbar and arm support, particularly during long drives.

- Scoot your seat close enough so that you aren't the "one-arm cool dude" whose seat is so far back that they strain their neck and shoulders to hold the steering wheel at arm's length. Your shoulders and neck should be relaxed.

- Don't hold the steering wheel in a white-knuckled death grip, which increases muscle tension. Your grip should be light but secure.

- Make sure the headrest is not forcing your head forward.
- Stop to take a break to move and stretch as often as you need.

Short Sheri and Her Simple Solutions

Every week I see someone like Sheri with head, neck, and jaw pain. Sheri is short and finds herself repeatedly extending her head and neck backward to look up at people, including her tall husband. She wears high heels to make herself taller, which further exaggerates the backward bending of her knees because she has loose joints. Her posture from the side looks like a zigzag, with her hips too far forward, shoulders too far back, and head too far forward. When Sheri sits, her feet don't touch the ground, so she finds herself slumping to reach the back of the chair or has to sit on the front edge, which quickly becomes uncomfortable. Her upper arms are short as well, and her arms do not reach the armrests, so her neck and shoulders never get to unload their weight when she sits for hours working at the computer. Sheri is tired of having neck pain and headaches and decides she is ready to replace hurtful habits with healthy ones. She gives away most of her high heels and finds some stylish and supportive alternatives she can be happy with. She learns to stand with her knees balanced in neutral instead of bent backward and adjusts her posture with the "quick fix" discussed earlier. When talking with her husband, they now sit down for lengthy discussions so she doesn't have to look up or adjust as the circumstances dictate. Sheri wraps old phone books in duct tape to make footstools so her feet can touch the ground when she sits comfortably in the back of her computer chair and couch. Because Sheri's joints are loose, she makes an appointment with a physical therapist to help her establish an exercise program to improve the strength and stability of her joints. Sheri is feeling better and is on the road to healthier habits.

Working at the Computer

If you spend more than an hour a day on the computer, it is important for you to arrange your computer and workstation ergonomically. In

FIGURE 4.6: Twelve Tips for an Ergonomic Computer Workstation

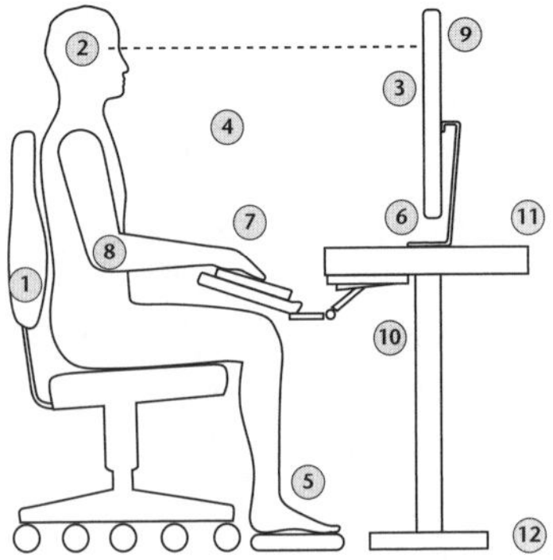

1. Use a good chair with a dynamic back and be sure to sit back in it. It is helpful if the chair is fully adjustable so you can customize it for you. Adjust the seat height, tilt, and back of the chair manually or add supports so you can maintain a balanced head and posture.

2. Make sure your eyes are in line with the screen, about 2–3 inches below the top of the computer monitor. If you have a newer monitor with less casing around the edges, the top of the viewing portion of the screen should be almost straight ahead, and the center of the screen should be about 17–18 degrees below that, as shown in the figure above.

3. Make sure there is no glare on the screen.

4. Sit at arm's length from the monitor, which should be centered and not turned at an angle.

5. Place your feet on the floor or on a footrest.

6. Use a document holder that is in-line with the screen. You may want to alternate sides occasionally so you are not always looking in the same direction.

7. Keep your wrists flat and straight. While wrist rests are popular, they can actually increase the pressure on the wrist.

8. Keep your arms and elbows relaxed and close to your body. Your elbows should be at a 90 degree (or slightly greater) angle. If you have armrests, they should be adjusted for your height and body type and should not interfere with your ability to move your elbows freely while you type and use the mouse.

9. Center the monitor/keyboard in front of you. Position your mouse so it is directly in front of your mouse hand and make sure your elbow is relaxed at your side, not resting on an armrest. The movement for the mouse should come from the elbow, and the arm should be relaxed. Many people place their mouse too far away and must strain to reach and use it. Sometimes when I use my laptop, I will use my mouse on my lap for a better position.

10. Use a negative or backward tilting keyboard or tray that is preferably adjustable in height.

11. Use a stable work surface.

12. Take frequent, short breaks (microbreaks). Remember to look 20 feet away for 2 seconds every 20 minutes. This is also a good time to stretch and move. Vary your activities so your body gets a break.

(Source: Text adapted from "12 Tips for an Ergonomic Computer Workstation." Illustration recreated with the kind permission of Professor Alan Hedge, PhD, CPE [http://ergo.human.cornell.edu].[23])

a recent case study, the pain level of a patient with neck and upper-extremity pain receiving physical therapy improved by 1, but when physical therapy was combined with addressing the causes and ergonomically arranging their work setting, the patient's pain level improved by 4.6.[22] The more time you spend on the computer, the more you will benefit from making smart and simple changes to alleviate the stress and strain on your head, neck, and jaw.

Remember that movement is essential to healthy joints and tissues, so change positions frequently and take microbreaks to move your body in the opposite directions. While writing this book, I have trained myself to use the mouse with both my left and right hands so I can break up the cumulative trauma of 10- to 12-hour days on the computer.

Put Perfect Posture into Practice:
How to Sleep

You spend about a third of your life sleeping. Getting a good night's rest is critical to your overall well-being and that of your head, neck, and jaw. Dr. William C. Dement, a pioneer in sleep medicine, has said, "We are not healthy unless our sleep is healthy."[24] Dr. Gilles J. Lavigne at the University of Montreal warns that a night of poor sleep will be followed by a day with more pain…and a day with a lot of pain will be followed by a night of poor sleep.[25] I currently use a full hour to problem-solve with patients. As we sort through and assess possible hurtful habits and their solutions, it becomes apparent that a lack of the right quantity and quality of sleep and the patient's sleeping position are frequently some of the biggest contributors to their pain and dysfunction.[26] "In fact, 90% of chronic pain patients reported that pain occurred before or at the onset of poor sleep."[27]

Paul: Invest in a Good Pillow

I worked with Paul, a wonderful older gentleman, who has suffered from neck pain for years. I introduced some stretches and postural training with some positive results. However, as soon as he switched to an orthopedic pillow and adopted good sleeping positions, his neck pain improved more than 50 percent. That is a great return on such a small investment.

Why does so much improvement result from such a small change? My opinion is that when you learn good sleeping habits and get enough sleep, you put your body into a healthy position so that it can rest and heal for about eight hours, or a third of your day. However, if you are in a hurtful position, you are likely damaging your body for the same extended period of time. And if you deprive yourself of the sleep you need, it is a bit like taking bread out of the oven before it is fully cooked.

In general, you should wake up feeling renewed. If you wake up feeling poorly, then more investigation is needed. Try the following ideas for a few weeks, and if you still experience little or no improvement, talk with your doctor about seeing a sleep specialist. Remember that no two people are the same and it can take time to change any habit, including your sleeping position. I will present guidelines and ideas that work for most people, but it is up to you—along with your health-care providers—to modify them to meet your individual needs.

Pick the Perfect Pillow

You can start by using a down-type pillow that you can mold into the right shape (see Figure 4.7) or an orthopedic pillow that supports the small curve of your neck. When you sleep on your side, you will need to fold your down pillow or get an orthopedic pillow with a wider portion on the side, because the distance from your ear to shoulder is almost double the distance needed to support the curve in your neck while lying on your back. If you are on your back, too many pillows or a pillow that is too large or too firm will push your head and jaw into an awkward posture. For a listing of the latest and greatest pillows my patients with jaw, neck, and head disorders have had success with, go to www.tmjhealingplan.com.

Wraparound pillows. If you sleep on your back and tend to roll your head to one side at night, you can wake up with a very stiff neck. You can place a pillow beside your head and rest your head against this in a neutral, balanced position or try wrapping the bottom edges of your pillow around the bottom of your neck and shoulder to create a type of cradle for your head to prevent rolling (see Figure 4.7a).

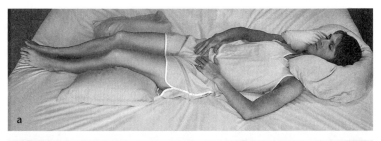

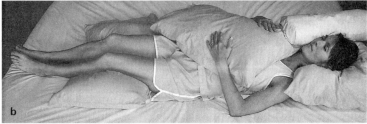

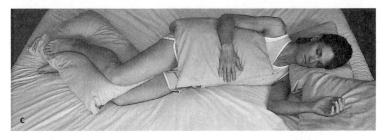

FIGURE 4.7: Balanced sleep positions: (a) molded neck pillow
wrapped around for support and pillow under knees,
(b) "psychological teddy bears" for stomach and side sleepers,
(c) side sleeping with pillow between knees and under upper arm

Cheek pillows and other psychological teddy bears. Most of us
have come to associate certain things with sleep. For example, many
side and stomach sleepers want to feel something against their face
(see Figure 4.7b). They are accustomed to having the pillow or bed
pressing on the side of their face, and this may even be a signal that
helps them go to sleep. If you switch your position to your back and
can't sleep without this sensation, try to substitute a blanket or small
pillow and set it gently next to your cheek while you are lying on your
back. Make sure you can breathe freely and that there is no pressure
on your jaw. Stomach sleepers who switch to their back may be more

comfortable with the transition if they place a pillow on their stomach. There may also be other situations, but you get the idea.

Body pillows. A body pillow can be helpful if you have previously been a stomach sleeper. Place a body pillow on the side you tend to roll over on. It will act a bit like a fence and can help stop you from rolling all the way over onto your stomach.

Use a Good Mattress. There is no "one-size-fits-all" mattress. You need to find a mattress that will support your spine and body in a balanced, neutral position and that is comfortable for you. Everyone is a little different, so try it before you buy it. If you sleep an average of eight hours each night, you'll spend about 2,920 restorative hours a year on it. Make sure it comes with a 30-day return policy, just in case. I have had patients spend thousands of dollars on mattresses that made them miserable.

Sleep on Your Back

Start your night by sleeping on your back with a pillow under your knees. Clinically, lying on your back with your knees slightly bent puts less pressure on your back, and I have found this position to be easier on the head, neck, and jaw muscles and joints. There are lots of possible variations—one knee bent on the pillow, one straight under the pillow, etc. The key is to be balanced. I prefer to rest my elbows at my side and my hands on my pelvis or thighs. This puts my shoulders in a healthy position. Stomach sleepers who are trying to kick the habit often feel much better with a pillow on their tummy they can hold and even one next to their face, which recreates the sensation of having their face and belly on the bed.

While on your back, you need a pillow for your head that supports the normal curve of your neck without pushing your head forward. Remember, big pillows or too many pillows cause a forward posture while sleeping that can strain your neck and make you more likely to clench or grind your teeth and swallow incorrectly. Proper support allows you to be in a good, balanced posture while you sleep.

If you want to stay on your back, but need some variety, try this suggestion. I came up with this idea after a surgery that forced me to sleep on my back for weeks. When I needed a change of positions, I would place a pillow along one side of my body and lie back on it so I was partially on my side, but still mostly on my back. It was just enough to help me feel a change of positions but not break the rules. Then I could switch sides. Keep in mind that sleeping on your back is not always the best position for everyone. My heavier patients tend to have difficulty breathing while flat on their back, and one of my patient's jaws would lock every time she lay flat, so work with your doctors to customize this healing plan for you.

Do not sleep with your arm or arms over your head or hand under your chin. These positions can strain the neck and shoulder muscles and create a common cause of pain and dysfunction in these areas. Likewise, bending an arm up to have your hand by your face all night will irritate your muscles and can adversely place pressure on your jaw. If you want something next to your face, try a soft pillow or blanket instead.

Try elevating the head of the bed. This elevation can help with reflux and certain trigger points. It sometimes helps patients who snore or feel uncomfortable while lying flat. Elevate the head-end part of the bed frame with very stable blocks up to 3–3½ inches high. Patients have gone to lumber stores or construction sites and asked for scraps of wood that they could duct tape together.[28] Many people try to sleep in recliners to elevate their head.

Sleep on Your Side

Although sleeping on your back is usually best for your muscles, you may have a health concern that prevents you from sleeping this way. If you fall into this category, the next best option is to sleep on your side. If you have a serious head, neck, and jaw problem, you generally should try to stay on your back. Sleeping on your side can put more pressure on your jaw, neck, and the shoulder you are lying on. If you must sleep on your side, it will take extra effort to be balanced because you have more variables to control. If possible, you should alternate sides. Most side sleepers I work with that are having troubles tend to sleep almost exclusively on one side, and we are often able to trace back many of their symptoms and postural problems to this sleeping position.

Level Your Head

On your side, you need a thick pillow or support. The distance from your head to the outside of your shoulder that needs to be spanned in order to allow you to level your head while sleeping on your side is much greater than the distance to the small curve in your neck that you need to support when lying on your back. Men and women with broad shoulders may need even more support. Many orthopedic pillows build this additional support into their design. However, if you use a down pillow or towel, you must remember to fold it in half in order to create the extra support you would need when sleeping on your side.

Do not to let your pillow push on your lower jaw. Instead, the bulk of the pressure should be on your cheek or head, providing gentle support to the jaw.

Level and Balance Your Spine and Extremities

Place a pillow between your knees and ankles when you lie on your side. This puts your hips, spine, and pelvis into a balanced position and can help prevent you from rolling onto your stomach (see Figure 4.7c on page 57).

Avoid curling up in the fetal position. This brings your head too far forward and can cause you to clench your teeth and swallow incorrectly.

Place a pillow under your upper arm (the one you aren't lying on) and in front of you. This puts your shoulder, neck, and wrist in a more relaxed position and helps prevent you from bringing your arm across your body and rounding your shoulders all night. It also helps limit your ability to roll onto your stomach or curl up in the fetal position (see Figure 4.7c on page 57).

Place a pillow under your trunk. If there is too much pressure on the shoulder you are lying on, try placing a thin towel or pillow under your trunk that leaves a hole or pocket for your shoulder. If you sleep exclusively on your side or have broad shoulders or shoulder problems, this will not only unload or take weight off your shoulder and neck, but will also level the spine. Try it. It is really quite comfortable and would be worth the effort if you sleep exclusively on your side.

Keep your wrists in a neutral position. It is not uncommon for people to bend their wrists during the night, which can irritate the carpal tunnel area. A pillow under the upper arm can help keep your wrist in a level, neutral position.

Avoid Sleeping on Your Stomach

I saw a young lady last week who was a stomach sleeper and had worn down her entire mandibular condyle and yet continued to sleep on her stomach.

Stomach sleeping is not an option for head, neck, and jaw pain sufferers. I don't encourage any of my patients to sleep on their stomachs. If you sleep on your stomach, you typically force your neck into extreme rotation, and then you rest the weight of your heavy head on your jaw all night. This places extreme pressure on the jaw and neck joints and irritates the joints and muscles. I have known patients who wake up with a dislocated jaw or herniated disk in their neck after sleeping on their stomach. Stomach sleeping can also cause back, hip, and shoulder pain. Stomach sleeping is a hard habit to break, but doing so is an essential step in reducing your pain and improving your function.

Many of my patients who have always slept on their stomachs have had success using pillows to create a type of fence to help prevent them from rolling onto their stomachs. Some people have actually sewn a small ball into the front of their pajamas to make rolling onto their stomach too uncomfortable. Be creative, but also be wise.

Change Unconscious Sleeping Habits

When my children were small and not sleeping through the night, I was introduced to the "magic" sleep book: Dr. Ferber's *Solve Your Child's Sleep Problems*.[29] Pediatrician Richard Ferber is the director of the Center for Pediatric Sleep Disorders at Children's Hospital in

Boston. His premise that applies here is that you partially wake several times throughout the night, and if everything is the way you feel it is supposed to be, you go back to sleep and don't even realize you ever woke up. However, if your covers are off or your pillow is on the floor, you will wake enough to pick up your pillow or pull up the covers and then go back to sleep.

As you begin to change your sleeping posture habits, you may wake to find you aren't in a healthy position. As in Dr. Ferber's example, you can use these partial waking moments to put yourself back into a healthy sleeping position before going back to sleep. It usually takes a week or two, but it may take longer for a new, healthier position to feel right. However, it is well worth it!

Other Helpful Sleep Tips

You will feel and function better if you get the right quantity and quality of sleep. This is so important that I would like to share a few more ideas to improve your salubrious slumber:[30]

- Establish a routine:
  - Go to bed at the same time each night and get up at the same time each morning.
  - Schedule yourself enough sleep time. Most people need seven to nine hours each night.
  - Wind down with the same routine to signal your body it is time to sleep.

- To prevent having to get up at night:
  - Avoid drinking all liquids one hour before bedtime.
  - Drink no alcohol three hours before bed.
  - Avoid caffeine six to eight hours before bedtime.

- To help you fall asleep:
  - Go to bed when you are tired.
  - Wind down with a relaxation CD (if needed).
  - Turn off the lights, reduce noise, and adjust the temperature to suit you.
  - Avoid stimulating activities late in the evening like using the computer and exercise.

- Regular exercise can help you sleep better, but exercise no later than two to three hours before going to bed.

• Avoid cool air blowing on you at night, which can aggravate sensitive muscles and joints.

• When you travel, bring your neck pillow and use the same sleep routines.

• A short nap in the middle of the day, even fifteen to twenty minutes, can help you feel alert and refreshed, but long or late naps might make it difficult for you to fall asleep at night.

• Use sleeping pills as a last resort.

Most everyone has trouble sleeping at one time or another, but if you've tried these tips and still regularly wake up feeling tired or are very sleepy during the day, you should probably see a doctor or sleep specialist. Identifying and addressing the cause of your sleep disturbances are critical in helping you feel and heal your best.[31]

Many people read and watch TV in bed. While it is best to use the bed primarily for sleep, those of you who do these things in bed should try these suggestions:

• When reading in bed, do not put pillows under your head. Instead, bring the book to you (see Figure 4.8).

• When watching television in bed, make sure the screen is directly in front of your line of vision and not too high or too low or at an awkward angle.

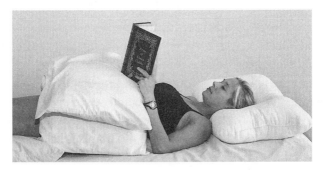

FIGURE 4.8: Balanced posture for reading in bed

Snoring and Sleep Apnea Can Be a Concern

Have you ever been told you snore or have trouble breathing at night? Snoring and sleep apnea are commonly associated with TMJ disorders and other chronic pain syndromes and may be an indication that your airway is obstructed. It could be that your tonsils are enlarged or your sinuses are blocked, which can also cause you to breathe through your mouth. You can often eliminate snoring by sleeping on your side, losing weight, and avoiding alcohol near bedtime. However, if your snoring is loud, frequent, and accompanied by shallow or stopped breathing, you may have sleep apnea. According to the NIH, "Sleep apnea is a common disorder that can be serious. In sleep apnea, your breathing stops or gets very shallow. Each pause in breathing typically lasts 10 to 20 seconds or more. These pauses can occur 20 to 30 times or more an hour."[32] If you aren't breathing, you are not taking in any oxygen and must wake up to start breathing again. This disturbs your sleep so you don't wake up feeling rested, and it can exacerbate your pain and dysfunction. Sleep apnea can be caused by a stuffy nose or a blocked air pipe. Sometimes the brain may "forget" to send a message to breathe. Some believe obstructive sleep apnea is caused by the inability of the mandible or lower jaw to keep the airway open and that people can find relief by using an intraoral device made by a specially trained dentist to maintain the airway.[33] Whatever the cause, if you experience sleep apnea or snore routinely, it is important to be evaluated by a specialist.

Summary

Good posture is paramount, whether we are sleeping, sitting, or standing. Most people know that driving a car with a flat tire is not only dangerous but can also throw off the alignment of the car and cause the tires to wear out unevenly. Yet we don't give a second thought to the importance of good alignment and postures for our bodies when we slouch, have a leg-length discrepancy, or park our bodies for the night in hurtful positions. You can help keep your body in alignment with this five-point inspection:

1. Establish a balanced sleeping position, preferably on your back, but the next best position is on your side. Get the pillows and supportive items you need to be successful.

2. Set up the places where you sit the most so that you can support the normal curves of your spine, unload the weight of your shoulders and arms, and make sure your feet can rest comfortably on a stable surface or footrest. This would include the couch, car, computer chair, and so forth.

3. Stand smart. Use the string analogy to help you focus on elongating and balancing your spine, head, and neck. Stand with your weight equally distributed on both legs.

4. Ergonomically arrange your work surface or computer area. The more time you spend doing an activity, the more important it is that you are in a balanced posture while doing it.

5. Identify and address any alignment problems, like a leg-length discrepancy, with the appropriate health-care specialist.

6. Make yourself a personalized checklist for change. Use the sample in Table 4.1 as a guide.

Table 4.1: Checklist for Change: Improving Posture

HURTFUL HABIT	HEALTHY HABIT	CHECKLIST FOR CHANGE
I sleep on my stomach or left side with my arm up under my pillow.	I will sleep primarily on my back and alternate sides if I need to, with my arm down.	I will keep my arm down. I will buy a good neck pillow that supports back and side postures. I will place a pillow under my knees and under my upper arm, with a body pillow next to me or sew a ball into the front of my pj's to help prevent me from rolling onto my stomach. I will start in a good position and correct whenever I wake.

(cont'd.)

Table 4.1: Checklist for Change: Improving Posture (cont'd.)

HURTFUL HABIT	HEALTHY HABIT	CHECKLIST FOR CHANGE
I slouch when I sit and my feet don't touch the ground.	I will sit in a good posture, with my head, neck, and jaw balanced and my feet supported.	I will add the appropriate lumbar support to my computer chair, car seat, and I will use pillows on the couch. I will tape together old phone books as footrests for use at the computer chair and while on the couch.
I am double-jointed and stand with my knees buckled backward, love wearing high heels, and like to stand with my weight on one leg.	I will stand with neutral knees and a balanced posture.	I will place sticky note reminders to check my posture. I will toss my high heels and replace them with cute and healthy alternatives. I will give my friends a nickel every time they catch me standing on one leg.

5

Step 3: TLC
Teeth Apart, Lips Together, and Calm Your Muscles and Mind

Your teeth should hardly ever touch. Even when you chew, you have food between your teeth. Yes, your back teeth may touch when you swallow, but gently, if at all, is better for your joints. When your jaw is in a resting position (it never completely rests), the general rule is "teeth apart, lips together." This rule is represented by the **TLC** in PoTSB TLC, and we will discuss some of the effects teeth can have on your jaw joints in this chapter.

The Harm of Teeth Touching

In one study, people with jaw muscle and joint pain held their teeth together 80 percent of the time, compared with 20 percent of the time for people who did not have pain.[1] If you clench or grind your teeth, do you clench because of the pain or did the clenching come first? The jury is still out, but experts suspect that people affected by TMJ disorders are less aware than most about the position of their teeth, which would make it harder for them realize when they are clenching or grinding.

What is the matter with your teeth touching? Here are some of the harmful results:

1. Your teeth touching can add wear and tear to your jaw joints.
   You may remember that a male can bite with a force of up to 266

pounds of pressure,[2] which is about the weight of some refrigerators, so your jaw can produce tremendous amounts of force, and as soon as your teeth touch, this force is transferred to your jaw joint. This added pressure can lead to early deterioration or arthritis of the TMJs.

2. Grinding your teeth or holding them together can squeeze important synovial fluid out of the disks in your jaw joint. It also can make the disks stick to the top of your mandibular condyles, which hinders their proper function.

3. Muscle pain and fatigue can occur when the muscles must tighten to keep the teeth together. This makes the muscles work harder than they need to. Muscle activity levels, as measured by the amount of electrical activity in these muscles, is two to three times higher when the teeth touch than when the teeth are not touching.[3]

4. It ruins your teeth. If you clench and grind, your teeth can wear down and even break. People who regularly clench and grind can wear down their teeth until their teeth are all the same height. Some teeth are so worn that the outer enamel of the tooth is gone and you can see the dentin, which is the next, somewhat yellowish, layer inside the tooth.

Bracing, Clenching, and Grinding

It is fairly easy to spot people who clench and grind their teeth. For many, their muscles are so tight and tense that they barely open their mouth when they talk. Their chewing muscles are often enlarged. You can often see their teeth touching at rest and when they speak. Their canine teeth are usually flat and all their teeth may be the same height. They often complain about headaches and jaw pain.

If you wake up in the morning with a headache or face, jaw, or tooth pain, there is a good chance you are grinding or clenching your teeth during the night. You may also be sleeping in a hurtful position. There are three general categories of teeth tension habits to become aware of and change:

Muscle Bracing

Muscle bracing occurs when you hold tension in the muscles that move the jaw for a prolonged period of time, but your teeth do not actually touch. Many of you may be thinking "my teeth are not touching," and yet your muscles are tense, tight, and overworked. Most people who brace their jaw muscles don't recognize what they are doing. They have held tension in those muscles for so long that they do not know how to relax them. Yet, bracing can produce the same level of tension as clenching your teeth together; that is, two to three times more tension than normal. A trained specialist can often tell if you brace by considering the following:

- You have little or no wear on your teeth.
- Your muscles are tense and taut when pressed.
- You are not conscious of clenching or grinding your teeth during the day.

Clenching

Clenching occurs when the muscles are tense and the teeth are touching. This is sometimes hard to recognize and many people are unaware that they clench. With clenching, the teeth are usually not ground down, as often occurs with grinding. Nevertheless, clenching still subjects the TMJs to a tremendous amount of unnecessary pressure and abuse.

Clenching is thought to be primarily caused by stress; however, a forward head posture can also set the stage for clenching. As soon as you bring your head forward, your teeth tend to come together. If you clench, you may be able to feel a bite line in your own mouth by sweeping your tongue along the inside of your cheek. If you feel a horizontal line along the inside of your cheek where your teeth come together, there is a good chance you are clenching or grinding.

Grinding

Grinding is also called bruxism. Some people grind their teeth so often at night that their teeth are flattened to the same height or grooved. Others grind their teeth so badly that they crack, loosen, or even chip their teeth. As with bracing and clenching, many people don't recognize they are grinding since they typically grind when they are sleeping. If something is not done to stop the damage, grinding can lead to damage of the jawbone, difficulties with the jaw muscles, and even loss of teeth.

Grinding peaks at age twenty, with the lowest occurrence at age seventy. Caffeine intake doubles the incidence of grinding. Other risk factors include smoking, medications such as antidepressants, sleep apnea, and xerostomia (dry mouth).[4]

Grinding your teeth at night can tighten and irritate your muscles and make you more likely to clench your teeth and keep tension in your muscles throughout the day. This can lead to an ongoing cycle of irritation and pain. Grinding primarily occurs when you sleep and is often associated with sleep apnea, which also occurs more often when sleeping on your back. Sixty percent of people who grind complain of poor sleep quality and quantity. The pain from grinding often wakes them during the night.

What You Can Do to Stop Bracing, Clenching, and Grinding

Just as the causes of clenching are multifaceted and still being discovered, so are the treatments. I will first discuss some of the potential causes and contributing factors and then review treatments that are safe, simple, and cost-effective to try. I will briefly discuss mouth guards or appliances and medications, which are probably the most common treatments.

Correct Your Posture and Tongue Position, and Get Enough Quality Sleep

Start with your posture. As soon as your head comes forward, your teeth tend to touch and your tongue wants to push against your teeth. So correcting your posture, as we discussed in Chapter 4, and training your tongue to rest on the roof of your mouth, as discussed in Chapter 6, are essential in terms of setting the stage for you to keep your teeth apart. Be sure to correct your posture when standing, sitting, and sleeping:

1. **Standing.** Pretend your head is being pulled by a string that is elongating your body toward the ceiling, anchor your tongue on the roof of your mouth, and distribute your weight evenly so your head can remain balanced.

2. **Sitting.** Use back supports if necessary to maintain a balanced head in relation to the normal curves in your spine. Try sitting up straight. If your teeth are apart and you look down, your teeth clench together. Place your tongue on the roof of your mouth, as this helps your jaw muscles relax.

3. **Sleeping.** Posture counts at night, too. If you sleep with two or three pillows under your head, curl up on your side in the fetal position, or sleep on your stomach with your head twisted to one side, your teeth will most likely come together. This sets the stage for you to clench and grind your teeth all night. (See sleeping postures in Chapter 4.) Because sleeping on your back can increase the likelihood of grinding, try elevating the head of the bed by putting a solid support under the headboard only. Alternatively, sleep on your side, with a pillow between your knees, using good posture as discussed in Step 2, also in Chapter 4.

   It is vital for you to get the right quality and quantity of sleep. Sixty percent of people who grind their teeth at night report poor sleep quality and often wake with pain. Some researchers believe that stress disrupts the quality and quantity of your sleep, which in turn could cause you to grind your teeth. Stress management is thus important in alleviating this cycle and is discussed in Chapter 11. Sleep apnea is also a risk factor for tooth grinding.[5]

Some Common Drugs Cause Clenching

Evaluate any medications you might be taking. Look for side effects that might contribute to any symptoms you are concerned about. For example, selective serotonin reuptake inhibitors (SSRIs) are commonly prescribed to treat depression, anxiety, obsessive-compulsive disorder, and post-traumatic stress disorder. However, side effects of these drugs include clenching, headaches, dizziness, and gastrointestinal difficulties. There are more than thirty medications in this category, including Prozac, Zoloft, Lexapro, and Paxil. If you use SSRIs, these medications may contribute to your symptoms. The agents fluoxetine and paroxetine seem to cause bruxism at night and are not recommended.[6] You may want to talk with your prescribing doctor and pharmacist about these symptoms and possible options.

Get Enough Folic Acid

According to Travell and Simons, grinding can sometimes be influenced by a restless muscle due to folic acid deficiency.[7] This can be similar to what happens in restless leg syndrome, but in this case it is in the jaw. So in addition to eating a healthy diet, you may want to be sure to get enough folic acid. According to the National Institutes of Health Office of Dietary Supplements, the average person fourteen years or older should have 400 micrograms of folate a day. Pregnant women need 600 micrograms. You can access this information at http://ods.od.nih.gov/factsheets/folate.asp.

Use an Alarm

Set your alarm to go off every hour during the day and check to see if your jaw is tense or your teeth are together. If they are, stop whatever you are doing. Consciously calm and relax your muscles and mind. First, let your jaw relax open, put your tongue on the roof of your mouth, and close your lips. Your tension should be gone, and you are on the road to replacing a hurtful habit with a healthy one. You will be checking the position of your teeth when you do your PoTSB TLC checks throughout the day.

Create a Buddy System

My husband used to grind his teeth at night. The noise would wake me up and I, in turn, woke him up to let him know he was grinding. This interruption stopped the grinding and allowed him to readjust into a better sleeping position so that after just a couple of weeks of serious effort, he stopped grinding his teeth at night. You can try the buddy system, either at night or during the day.

Calm and Relax Your Muscles and Mind

Stress, both physical and psychological, can increase the tension in your body and cause you to brace, clench, or grind. Some researchers believe these habits are caused by the central nervous system gone awry. Pain is an example of a physical stress that can cause you to clench. Danger is an example of a psychological stress. When we don't feel safe, we trigger our body's sympathetic nervous system, which tenses our muscles in preparation for a fight-or-flight response. Establish safe surroundings and relaxed relationships. Ways to reduce stress are discussed in Step 9 of Chapter 11. You need to have a stress-management plan and techniques that work for you to calm and relax your muscles and mind. At Canyon Rim Physical Therapy, many of our patients have been able to improve their ability to relax their jaws and calm their minds with jaw-specific relaxation exercises, breathing techniques, and the use of visualization and relaxation CDs. Go to www.tmjhealingplan.com for suggestions.

Kick These Hurtful Habits

- Stop smoking.

- Decrease or eliminate caffeine. (Check labels carefully because caffeine is a common ingredient, even in so called "decaffeinated" coffee and drinks.)

- Get help if you have sleep apnea or xerostomia (dry mouth).

Your Teeth and the Impact of a Bad Bite

According to the *Harvard Health Letter*, in the 1970s and 1980s the school of thought regarding TMJ disorders was that jaw pain was a result of a jaw joint problem caused by a bad bite. And to alleviate the problem, the bite and jaw joints needed to be "fixed." Unfortunately, this resulted in many unnecessary and irreversible treatments such as crowns, grinding down of teeth, and lots of jaw-joint surgeries. While all of these procedures certainly have their appropriate place, in the last 10 years medical thinking has changed.[8]

We now know that pain and dysfunction of the jaw muscles and soft tissues are the most common causes of TMJ-related problems. The NIH pleads with consumers to first explore their safe reversible options, many of which we have tried to educate you about in this book, before undergoing irreversible procedures. Also, keep in mind that since your teeth should never touch except momentarily when you swallow, the impact of a nonperfect bite is lessened if you can get your PoTSB TLC in order, which will help you keep your teeth slightly apart. If your bite is "off" or causing you problems, keep in mind that the muscles or jaw joint problems may be the true cause of the malocclusion or bad bite. Physical therapy, appropriate exercises, and jaw appliances or splints are a few of the less intrusive options that can help address these concerns and restore balance.

What Is a Jaw Appliance or Splint?

There are many types of jaw appliances or splints, otherwise known as *intraoral occlusal orthotics appliances*. According to a recent report published in the *New England Journal of Medicine*, the most common jaw appliances are custom-made of a hard acrylic and are similar to retainers that you can easily insert and remove from your mouth. They typically fit over the upper or lower teeth. Splints can be helpful for many aspects of TMJ dysfunction. According to the report, these appliances are designed to:

- improve the function of the jaw joint or TMJ by changing the joint mechanics and increasing potential mobility or movement.

- improve the function of the chewing muscles while reducing abnormal muscle function.

- protect your teeth if you grind and clench your teeth.

- increase the person's awareness of hurtful oral habits and possibly help alter the "central motor system areas that initiate and regulate masticatory function."[9]

Mouth guards are different. They are typically not custom-made. They are soft and flexible and fit over the teeth to protect them and other structures in the mouth from the damage caused by trauma in contact sports or from clenching or grinding your teeth. Mouth guards are usually only worn at night or while playing sports. Try not to bite on your mouth guard, splint, or any other appliance you may be using. Your teeth may be better protected from the abuse, but it typically still can adversely affect your jaw joints.

Who Needs a Splint and What Should a Good Splint Do?

A splint is not necessary for everyone with TMJ disorders and much research is still needed. In 2004 the Cochrane Collaboration did a literature review on occlusal splints. The group felt there was insufficient evidence to either support or refute the use of oral-appliance therapy.[10] However, according to a 2008 *New England Journal of Medicine* report, "These devices may play a role in alleviating the pain and dysfunction of temporomandibular disorders in 70–90% of patients."[11]

There are a multitude of splints and appliances available and many reasons for wearing them. According to TMJ experts Mariano Rocabado and Z. Annette Iglarsh there are two primary functions of splints:[12]

- A splint or jaw appliance should help to relax muscles that are out of balance by allowing the jaw to close in its most relaxed position and improve hurtful habits. This should help relieve symptoms that are caused by TMJ dysfunction and put your jaw into a physiological position of rest. This is the position in which your jaw is the most relaxed and functions best. You should eventually feel your muscles relax and your pain and symptoms should improve. A good splint may take a little getting used to, but it should not make your symptoms worse and should help you stop clenching. Clenching or grinding your teeth may have moved them out of alignment. By maintaining your jaw in the correct position, your teeth can move into a more optimal position as well. According to Rocabado and Iglarsh, this program of relaxation can improve function in thirty to ninety days.

- Splints are also used to help alleviate problems with the inner workings of the joint. Technically, this condition is called an *internal derangement of the TMJ* and might include problems with the disk, such as problematic clicking and a history of locking. For example, people who have a history of their jaw locking but who are able to unlock their jaw may have a splint made to help keep the joint in a stable position so it won't keep locking and can be in a better position to heal. A good splint can also help reduce inflammation and pain in the jaw joints, reduce the risk for additional bone loss, and help protect the teeth.

Typically, an appliance alone will not solve your TMJ problem, but a jaw appliance that is balanced and made correctly can help provide an environment for your jaw to improve. Splints are most successful when used in conjunction with other treatments and when addressing and eliminating hurtful habits like those discussed in this book. Conversely, a splint that is not made correctly or one that is worn inappropriately can be deleterious.

Train Your Tongue

Training your tongue to rest on the roof of your mouth (discussed in Chapter 6) is absolutely critical in helping to relax your jaw muscles and keep your teeth apart. Don't miss this simple but essential step.

Lips Together

In order to keep your teeth apart and muscles calm and relaxed, you need your tongue to be resting up on the roof of your mouth. However, if you think about it, what keeps your tongue up on your palate against gravity? The answer is gentle suction, or as Rocabado and Iglarsh would call it, "negative air pressure." But you can only maintain this suction if your lips are closed. As soon as you part your lips, you lose suction. This can be a huge obstacle for someone with a short upper lip, which is very common in people who have been mouth breathers instead of nose breathers. You can usually tell if someone has a short upper lip, because at rest their lips are separated and you can see their teeth (as seen in the first photo of Figure 5.2 on page 79). If the lips are together as they should be, you will not see any teeth, only lips. Correcting this is not easy, because you must first eliminate the cause, which may be allergies or a nasal obstruction. You must be able to breathe through your nose so you can keep your lips sealed. However, you will likely need to stretch and retrain your upper lip to its new length and position. Then you will have more success with keeping your tongue on the roof, because you can now maintain the gentle suction needed to do so, which in turn allows you to separate your teeth and relax your jaw muscles. These steps are all interrelated.

Retraining for TLC: Teeth Apart, Lips Together, and Calm Muscles and Mind

All exercises and activities should be symptom-free: No pain, grinding, clicking, locking, or catching should occur.

General Exercises and Activities

Eventually you will do the PoTSB TLC exercises several times a day to bring yourself to a home base of healthy head, neck, and jaw postures that should better enable the relaxation of your jaw muscles and the separation of your teeth. Since we have not yet introduced all of the concepts, let me briefly introduce a few pieces.

EXERCISE \ *Three Steps to Tongue Up, TLC, and Breathe Deep*

1. **Tongue Up.** Start in a good posture or position. For deep relaxation, let your jaw completely relax and allow your mouth to hang open. With all of your tension gone, put your tongue in a resting position on the roof of your mouth and focus on your tongue at rest. (This step is described more fully in Chapter 6.) Now add step 2.

2. **TLC.** Teeth apart, lips together, and calm the muscles and mind. Now, keeping your teeth slightly apart, gently close your lips. (If your upper lip is short, it may be uncomfortable for you to keep your lips closed. You may want to try the additional exercises at the end of this chapter to stretch your upper lip). Remember, you should have your tongue on the roof of your mouth, your teeth should be slightly apart, your lips together, and your jaw and neck muscles should be calm and relaxed.

3. **Now breathe through your nose (you have to if your lips are closed), expanding your diaphragm.** Your lower ribs and belly should expand and contract (which is discussed more fully in Step 5 of Chapter 7). A more relaxed jaw will result. If this position feels new to you, it may take time and much awareness to change these habits.

EXERCISE \ *Orbiting*

This exercise was described by Rocabado and helps control the movement of the TMJs.[13] Orbiting can gently relax, unwind, and help retrain muscles that brace, clench, and grind and that are out of balance. This gentle movement and stretching help these muscles relax. This can break the pain cycle and get you on the road to recovery. This exercise is simple, but it is one of the most powerful exercises I have found for TMJ health. Therefore, we will be revisiting it in many chapters. Do not do these exercises if there is any possibility your jaw may be "locked" or you may have another serious joint dysfunction. Do you have any popping or clicking noises in the jaw? As always, if you have any questions, check with a TMJ expert first.

1. Start with the front third of your tongue on the roof of your mouth, in resting position and teeth slightly apart.

2. Gently open and close your mouth in the pain-free range while keeping your teeth apart (see Figure 5.1).

   Rocabado recommends doing six repetitions of this exercises six times per day. However, the frequency and method depends on your individual needs. If I simply had tight jaw muscles, this could be a great exercise to actively move, stretch, and relax them, and I would do them as needed.

3. You can use a mirror with this exercise to help retrain and ensure that your nerves and muscles learn to open vertically straight. Many people with TMJ disorders have a learned "limp," and their jaw will deviate to one side as they open. It is easy to remember to do this exercise when you wash your hands and therefore likely have a mirror available.

   With your tongue anchored on the roof of your mouth, your jaw joint can rotate or orbit with less translation, or sliding, which can irritate the joint. This can replace unbalanced movement with healthy movement, which is critical to the well-being of every joint.

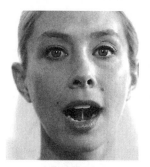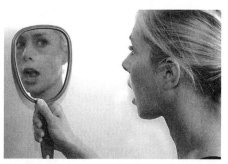

FIGURE 5.1: Orbiting with and without a mirror

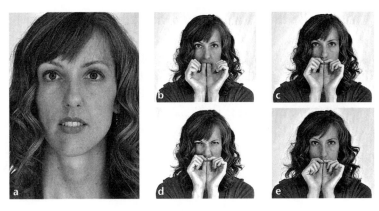

FIGURE 5.2: Short upper lip and Thumb-Pull Stretch

Stretches and Exercises for a Short Upper Lip

Talk with your provider about using the exercises below to help stretch your short upper lip so that you can keep your lips closed (see Figure 5.2a). Lip closure improves your tongue's ability to maintain gentle suction that will help keep your tongue on the roof and your teeth apart. It is important to stretch your upper lip first. If you try to strengthen it before getting the functional upper-lip length you need, it may cause a little muscle called the *mentalis* to put pressure on and crowd the lower teeth.[14] You no longer need to stretch your upper lip when it can comfortably rest and reliably maintain a seal with your bottom lip. Some recommend using a special tape that is safe for use on the skin and lips to actually hold your lips together. Other specialists make a mouth shield to help facilitate this stretching and retraining process. You may need the help of a specialist.

EXERCISE \ ***Thumb-Pull Stretch***

First, you will want to wash your hands or wear surgical gloves. Then, place your thumbs underneath your upper lip all the way to the top, directly underneath your nostrils (see Figure 5.2b). Hold your upper lip between your index fingers and thumbs and gently pull down toward the lower lip (see Figure 5.2c). You can add some resistance by wrinkling your nose (see Figure 5.4d). Hold for 10 seconds (see Figure 5.2e). Repeat 6 times. Do this several times a day as tolerated until you achieve enough length to maintain lip closure.[15]

EXERCISE \ *Rubber-Tubing or Cotton-Roll Stretch*

Place a piece of surgical rubber tubing (about ¼ inch thick and about 2½ inches long) or wet cotton rolls (i.e., like the rolls of cotton the dentist places in your mouth when you have dental work done) behind and under your upper lip horizontally under your nose. Leave the tubing or cotton there for up to four hours at a time. Don't ever swallow this roll, and you might want to remove it before you go on a date or have your picture taken.[16]

EXERCISE \ *Tape*

Physical therapists use special tapes for many purposes, but it wasn't until I was researching for this book that I was introduced to this idea. Followers of the Buteyko breathing method feel so strongly about breathing through the nose, they actually tape their client's mouths closed. They use a special 3M micropore mouth tape that is porous, easy to remove, and available at some pharmacies and medical supply shops. They place a small piece of this tape vertically over the lips from top to bottom. The tape could also provide a nice stretch for a short upper lip as well as a constant reminder to breathe through your nose. Buteyko teachers advocate the use of tape during the night and at any time possible during the day until you are able to maintain lip closure, which encourages breathing through your nose and with your diaphragm.[17] This is an idea that could be discussed with your health-care providers. I would talk to your doctor before using the tape, especially at night, as some patients with various sleep disorders may need to open or adjust their mouth to breathe and breathing is very important, even if it is through your mouth.

EXERCISE \ *Lips Together Strengthening Exercises*

If any of these exercises increase your symptoms, discontinue them and continue to work with your specialist to modify your approach to best meet your needs. After you have stretched your short upper lip to the appropriate length, you can strengthen its ability to maintain lip closure by using the following exercises:

Lip Press: You can simply press your lips together or you can add some variety with the button-and-string exercise that follows next.

Button: Put a large, clean button on a string. Hold the button inside your mouth, just behind your lips, with your lips together and the string outside of your mouth. Gently pull on the string, which forces your lips to stay pressed together to prevent you from pulling the button out of your mouth.[18]

Summary

You may have been surprised to learn that your teeth should only touch when you swallow. Learning to keep your tongue on the roof of your mouth and lips together can help you to relax your jaw and separate your teeth. Sometimes clenching may be beyond your control, but usually there are many things that can be done to help you overcome the hurtful habits of clenching and grinding and put your jaw into a healthy posture, including the following:

1. Your teeth are less likely to touch when your tongue is on the roof of your mouth and you establish the TLC habits of **T**eeth apart, **L**ips together, and **C**alming your muscles and mind. This is also a critical step to achieving correct swallowing, speech, and tongue positions.

2. Your lips need to be able to stay together to maintain the negative air pressure that allows your tongue to stay gently suctioned to the roof of your mouth. When your tongue is anchored on the roof, your jaw muscles can relax.

3. Remember, your teeth should only touch momentarily and lightly when you swallow.

4. Calm and relax your muscles and your mind. You also need to resolve any contributing factors such as getting enough sleep or discussing with your doctor any medications that may be contributing to your clenching or grinding. It is important to breathe through your nose and with your diaphragm.

5. Consider the use of an appropriate occlusal splint to help decrease your tension and grinding.

6. Make yourself a checklist for change. Use the following sample table as a guide.

Table 5.1: Checklist for Change: Teeth Apart, Lips Together

HURTFUL HABIT	HEALTHY HABIT	CHECKLIST FOR CHANGE
I clench my teeth during the day and grind my teeth at night.	TLC: Teeth apart, Lips together, and Calm my muscles and mind. I will get my tongue to rest on the roof of my mouth, which will help my jaw muscles relax and my teeth to separate.	I will rest my tongue on the roof of my mouth. I will ensure good sleeping posture and practice PoTSB TLC. I will talk to my doctor about my SSRI medications and their effect on clenching. I will listen to a relaxation imagery CD before bed. I will decrease my caffeine intake. I will think about a splint.
I can't keep my lips together because of a slightly short upper lip.	Lips together, teeth apart.	I will check with my TMJ expert. I will stretch my upper lip with thumb pull and tubing. After stretching is done, I will strengthen my ability to keep lips closed with button exercise.

6

Step 4: Train Your Tongue and Swallow Carefully

Your tongue is a much overlooked but very important muscle. It helps you taste, chew, and swallow a delicious meal; drink a beverage; and communicate with those around you. When your tongue is anchored and functioning correctly, it can help your head, neck, and jaw muscles relax and obtain the rest they need. If your tongue is so important, when was the last time you did a few tongue push-ups to keep it in shape? That may sound odd right now, but after you have read this chapter, I hope you will be motivated to tone and retrain your tongue.[1]

You use both your tongue and jaw when you swallow. You can't swallow correctly if your tongue is out of shape or out of balance. Many people with jaw problems swallow incorrectly, which can add additional stress to the jaw joints. Training your tongue and learning to swallow correctly involve changing subconscious habits. When was the last time you thought about the position of your tongue and teeth or how you swallow or breathe? If these habits are not healthy ones, you may be headed for trouble. As discussed earlier, hurtful oral habits are kind of like driving a car with one foot on the gas and the other slightly on the brake. You can still drive, but it is not efficient and you are going to quickly wear out your brakes. In this example, the brakes are like your jaw joints. If you have a tongue thrust and swallow abnormally, you will still be able to talk and swallow, but it can put undue wear and tear on your jaw joints and associated structures.

The Resting Position of the Mandible

Just as the posture of your spine is important, the posture, or position, of your mandible is vitally important to the well-being of your head, neck, and jaw. In the medical community, this healthy posture of your jaw is often referred to as the resting position of the mandible.

Tongue position is very important in the proper development of the palate and the function of your mouth and face in general. Professors Mariano Rocabado and Z. Annette Iglarsh have done much research in this regard, documenting the development of the mouth. Their book, *Musculoskeletal Approach to Maxillofacial Pain*, demonstrates how hurtful habits can have an especially profound impact during development.[2] There is also research with monkeys to demonstrate that changing the resting position of the tongue from where it is supposed to be on the roof of the mouth or having to breathe through the mouth adversely affected a monkey's bite and facial structure development.[3] I hope that these healthy habits will be taught to children so these important facial structures can develop appropriately.

Tongue on the Roof

Let's talk about the first **T** in PoTSB TLC, which stands for "tongue on the roof." Your tongue, teeth, and facial muscles dynamically balance each other, and when one is out of place or not working correctly, it throws off the balance or equilibrium of everything else. The first step is to figure out what hurtful habits you have, if any, and then start to make the necessary changes.

Assess Your Tongue Position

Let's begin with some testing. Sometimes the hardest part is getting a clear picture of what you actually do. Here are two tests you can try.

> EXERCISE \ *Where Is Your Tongue?*
>
> For this test, try to be in the posture or position you normally assume most of the time. Now, pay attention to where your tongue is resting. Is the tip of your tongue resting against the back of your front top or

bottom teeth? Make a note of where it rests. You may need to check yourself throughout the day to catch yourself when you may not be on your best behavior.

EXERCISE \ ***Does Your Tongue Tip Touch?***

Next, try a test used by many speech therapists and myotherapists (muscle therapists). Make note of what happens to the tip of your tongue as you say the letters *T, D, N, L, S,* and *Z?* Don't read any more until you try the test.[4]

Okay, did the tip of your tongue touch your front teeth at all? In the English language, if the tip of your tongue touches your front teeth when you say these letters or when it is at rest, then you most likely have a tongue thrust.

If you have a tongue thrust, don't panic! You are not alone and probably just need some tongue toning and training. It is estimated that 50 percent of normal eight-year-old children have a tongue thrust.[5] A tongue thrust occurs when the tip of the tongue pushes against the teeth when resting, talking, and/or swallowing. Other terms used to describe a tongue thrust relate to an abnormal swallow, such as reverse, atypical, or aberrant swallow. A tongue thrust can actually move your teeth and adversely affect your bite and jaw joints.[6] A tongue thrust is common in people with TMJ-related symptoms. I think one of the reasons so many people exhibit tongue thrust is because so many have poor posture. As we saw in Chapter 4, a forward head posture can alter the position of the jaw and its associated structures. A tongue thrust could also be a result of hurtful habits during development, like thumb sucking or the prolonged use of pacifiers.

Although many people exhibit a slight tongue thrust, others are much more severe. (Yes, I am warped by my education and am always watching people's tongues when they talk.) You can watch yourself in a mirror. Your tongue may push against the front top or bottom teeth while you talk; you may even see it poking out between your teeth. When speaking English, the only time the tip of your tongue should touch your front teeth is when you make the "th" sound, as in the words *thirsty* or *Thursday*.[7]

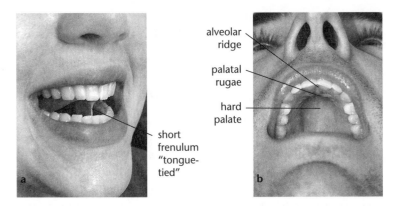

FIGURE 6.1: (a)"Tongue-tied" short frenulum and (b) hard palate, or roof of mouth, with upper alveolar ridge and palatal rugae

Anchoring on the "Spot"

You can usually eliminate a tongue thrust by toning and training your tongue to rest in the right spot. For the tip of the tongue, this spot is on or near the upper *alveolar ridge*, which is the roof of your mouth from where your top teeth insert to your hard palate. If you run the tip of your tongue along this area, you will feel lots of ridges or bumps called *palatal rugae* on the roof of your mouth just behind your top teeth but in front of the curved roof on the top of your mouth called the *hard palate* (see Figures 6.1b and Figure 6.2). These ridges or bumps give your tongue something to push off from and give your tongue traction in an otherwise slippery mouth when you swallow and speak. We sometimes refer to this ridge area as the "spot." When you pronounce the letters *T, D, N, L, S,* and *Z,* your tongue should touch on or near the upper alveolar ridge. I often have patients suction their tongue on the roof of their mouth to make a "cluck" sound in order to help them find this spot. Or you can place the front of your tongue on this ridge without touching your front teeth. Then, as you relax your tongue in its new home, it will splay, or expand, along the roof of your mouth, and the sides of your tongue may touch your teeth. However, the tip of your tongue should not touch your teeth at rest. Your tongue is longer than you may think and is anchored below to the *hyoid bone* (see Figure 6.2).

It may be helpful to think of your tongue as an anchor and your lower jaw or mandible as a boat floating on the water. For a ship's crew to really take a break, they have to drop anchor so they can be sure the boat will stay in the right place while they relax. However, they can't just drop the anchor anywhere. They have to find the right spot for it to take hold and stabilize the ship. The same is true for your jaw. For your jaw to take a break, you have to drop your tongue anchor, but you can't just drop it anywhere. You have to find "the spot."

You are probably wondering, if an anchor goes downward, how is your tongue supposed to rest when it is going up against gravity? That is a good question. Once you have a toned and trained tongue and teach it how to find "the spot," it will stay anchored with gentle suction that holds your tongue anchor in place. Your lips should remain closed to maintain this suction. This is the place your tongue should start to perform its important jobs, such as swallowing, and then return to and park on "the spot" afterward.

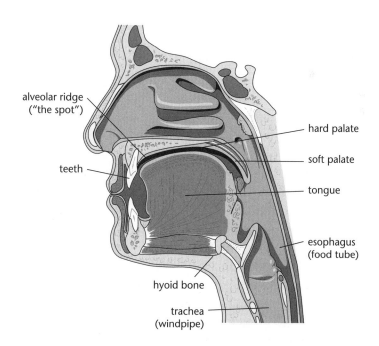

FIGURE 6.2: Side view of tongue, palate, and head

EXERCISE \ *Finding "the Spot"*

You can help your tongue find this healthy spot by making a clucking sound. Suction your tongue against the roof of your mouth and then release it. If you can make a good loud cluck, this is a good sign.

Positioning the Rest of Your Tongue

Now that you know where to put the tip of your tongue, what about the rest of it? The front, middle, and back of your tongue should rest on the palate. Speech-language pathologist Hilary Wilson describes how far back on the palate your tongue should touch. She says it should touch all the way from the place you make "T" on the alveolar ridge ("the spot") to where you pronounce "Ka, ka, ka" (as in Karate), near the back of the palate.[8] That represents about two-thirds of your tongue (see Figure 6.2 on page 87).

If you find you are having trouble anchoring your tongue on the roof of your mouth, it is usually due to a lack of tone. In other words, your tongue is out of shape. The exercises at the end of this chapter should help strengthen and train your tongue to be an anchor for the lower jaw.

Positioning Your Lips and Teeth

As you get your tongue into position, you need to seal your lips closed. With both lips sealed and your tongue anchored on the roof of your mouth, you create a negative air pressure and suction that help hold your tongue in place against gravity. With your tongue anchored to the roof and your lips sealed, the muscles of your craniomandibular system (your head, neck, and jaw) enter a reflex relaxation stage and the lower jaw can descend, or drop, to its resting position. This allows your muscles to relax and your teeth to rest slightly apart, creating what is called *freeway space* between your teeth. This is important if you clench or grind your teeth, and it can be helpful in patients with neck pain and headaches.[9]

If you have difficulty closing your lips or keeping them closed, you may have a short upper lip. This is often brought on by thumb sucking, extended use of a pacifier or bottle, or mouth breathing. If you can't close your lips, it changes the atmospheric pressure needed to maintain the gentle suction necessary to keep your tongue on the roof of your mouth. You may need to stretch your upper lip by doing the stretches for short upper lips outlined in Chapter 5 so you can eventually get your lips to seal comfortably together. With your lips sealed it will be easier to maintain the gentle suction needed to keep your tongue in place on the roof of your mouth.

Breathe Correctly

Placing your tongue on "the spot" simultaneously initiates other healthy habits, such as breathing through your nose. If you have a stuffy nose or allergies and have to take your tongue off the spot to open the airway so you can breathe, you will breathe the wrong way. When you are exerting energy, such as when you are running up the stairs or exercising, you may breathe for a short time through your mouth. Don't stress. As long as you aren't running up and down stairs 24/7, you should be okay. However, in a professional course taught by Canadian manual therapists, they shared that some Olympic athletes had significantly improved their times by learning to breathe nasal diaphragmatically with their tongues on "the spot" during their sports.[10] (We discuss breathing techniques in Chapter 7.)

Common Tongue Troubles

If you find it difficult to anchor your tongue on the roof of your mouth, you may have one of a number of troubles, including being tongue-tied, or having too large a tongue or too high a palate.

Tongue-Tied

You may have *ankyloglossia,* or be "tongue-tied." There is a membrane underneath your tongue that connects the floor of your mouth to the undersurface of your tongue, called the *frenulum.* If this connection is too short or tight, it can prevent the tip of your tongue from reaching "the spot" or prevent you from maintaining two thirds of your tongue on the roof with gentle suction.

You can see your frenulum and try to assess its length by looking in the mirror and trying to suction your tongue on the roof of your mouth like you are going to say "cluck," but then open your mouth keeping your tongue in this position. Your frenulum will stretch and look almost like a string underneath your tongue (see Figure 6.1a on page 86). If your frenulum is too short or tight you may not even be able to get your tongue to suction on the roof of your mouth. Gentle stretching can often elongate the frenulum enough to allow your tongue to reach and rest on the spot. If this is not sufficient, work with a TMJ expert or speech-language pathologist to find the best solution for you. Sometimes the frenulum needs to be clipped. A tied tongue is important to resolve because it can also impact proper speech and development, and even make it difficult to clean your teeth with your tongue after snacks. However, these problems are usually observed in only the more severe instances of ankyloglossia. Thus, it is important to note that each individual who is tongue-tied requires a thorough individual assessment and evaluation in order for the most appropriate management strategies to be selected.[11]

Large Tongue

You may have a tongue that is too large, which is called *macroglossia*. Speech-language pathologist Hilary Wilson reports that this condition is very rare.[12] It is much more common for someone to feel their tongue is too large because his or her tongue is out of shape. Often, people with large tongues have scalloping on the sides of their tongues, where their teeth and tongue interact. However, it can also occur in people who grind their teeth or suffer from sleep disorders like sleep apnea.[13] Wilson goes on to say that most people who complain of their tongue being too large lack strength throughout their entire tongue. While I thought this only happened in pirate movies, some doctors actually trim or cut a tongue that people feel is too large. Wilson reports this procedure can often be avoided by exercise and training. All reasonable conservative measures should be explored before doing something irreversible, such as going under the knife to cut your tongue.[14]

High Palate

Your palate may be too tall. Thumb suckers tend to develop a high palatal arch in the roof of the mouth. If the arch in your palate is too tall, you will be able to rest less of your tongue on the roof of your mouth. You will have to obtain suction from a smaller area near the front half of your tongue.

Tongue Toning and Training Exercises

Exercises should be pain-free and you should not do all of these exercises at one sitting. I generally recommend adding one or two new exercises at a time. Discontinue the exercises after your tongue is adequately toned and trained to rest on "the spot," and when you can speak and swallow correctly.

EXERCISE \ *Clucking*

Suction your tongue on the roof of your mouth. Then release your tongue, making a *cluck* sound. We mentioned this activity earlier as a way to help the tongue find its position and create suction on the roof of the mouth, but it can also be done as an exercise.

My youngest child still had a noticeable tongue thrust in elementary school, and one of the ways we practiced correcting his tongue position was by pretending we were chickens and making clucking sounds while we flapped our wings and waddled around the house to make the exercise more fun. You can try this, too. You can make many of your exercises lots of fun.

EXERCISE \ *Tongue Push-Ups*

Press your tongue up along the palate, or roof of your mouth. Hold it there for 10 to 20 seconds, then relax. Repeat this exercise 5 to 10 times, 2 to 3 times per day. To make this more exciting, you can try an exercise a first grader shared with me when I was teaching a group of school children. She was in speech therapy and said tongue push-ups could be made more fun by placing an easily dissolvable piece of cereal, like a Corn Flake or Cheerio, on the middle of your tongue and holding it up against the roof of your mouth in the correct position until the food dissolves. Eat five to ten pieces of cereal this way in the morning and five to ten in the evening.

Typically, I would have you do tongue push-ups with your lips closed. However, if you are trying to stretch your tongue, you can also do this exercise with your lips apart and mouth open, which works the back of your tongue to stretch the frenulum.

Remember to keep your tongue gently on the roof of your mouth even when you are not exercising.

EXERCISE \ *Stick Out Your Tongue*

I know your mom told you it wasn't nice to stick out your tongue at people, but sticking out your tongue can be a good exercise for toning and training your tongue, and some feel it helps ease muscle tension in the jaw and face. If you don't want to hurt anyone's feelings, do this exercise when you are alone, or better yet, get your friends to do the exercise with you. When you do this exercise, it is important to stick your tongue out straight for 3 to 5 seconds and then pull your tongue back in. Repeat 3 to 5 times. Point your tongue as if you are licking a sucker. It should be straight and flat like a board. Remember that even a simple exercise like this could potentially irritate someone with a serious jaw disorder. This is why we advise that all exercises be guided by your health-care providers.

EXERCISE \ *Sound and Speech Exercises*

Your tongue is important in speech, but it may not be working the right way when you speak. Here are some ways to check and strengthen different parts of the tongue. Remember, the tip of your tongue should not touch your front teeth when you speak English, except when you make the "th" sound, as when you say "Thursday."

- **Alveolar Consonants.** To strengthen the tip of the tongue going to the alveolar ridge, practice saying the alveolar consonants *T, D, N, L, S,* and *Z* that we used in the self-test. Try saying these words with added force: "Ted and Suzie love lollipops and salty donuts." You may notice that your tongue touches the ridge with all the letters except *S* and *Z* where it goes very close to the ridge but does not touch, in order to allow air to pass through the space to make the correct sounds.[15]

- **Jumping Chinchillas.** To strengthen the middle part of the tongue, say the sounds "ch" and "J" as in "Chinchillas cheat at checkers" and " Jump jam jars."

- **Kicking Gargoyles.** Saying the *K* and *G* sounds provide good exercises for the back, or posterior, part of the tongue. Practice words like "Kate kicked gagging gargoyles."

EXERCISE \ **Buttercup**

Finally, a good general speech exercise is to repeat the word "buttercup" quickly and succinctly. Clearness is more important than speed. This helps you to get front to back movement, which is important in normal tongue and oral functions, such as swallowing.

This exercise is sometimes used by speech-language pathologists to evaluate speech rate. Saying "buttercup" causes a front-to-back movement starting with the labial (lips) "bu," alveolar (near those ridges) "ter," and then palatal (roof of mouth near the back) "cup," with the "cu" being formed with the back of the tongue at the back of the palate.

Swallow Correctly

Now let's talk about the **S** in PoTSB TLC, which stands for "swallow correctly." Do you know how often you swallow every day? It may be hard to imagine, but you swallow approximately once every minute when you are awake, about eight times a minute when you eat, and much less when you are asleep.[16] Just for fun, let's see how that adds up if you sleep eight hours and swallow half as much as when you slumber. If you are awake 16 hours, then you get 960 waking swallows per day. But that's not all. When you eat, you swallow about eight times a minute. If you eat three 30-minute meals a day and one 10-minute snack, for 80 total minutes of eating, you can add 800 swallows to your day. However, you still swallow when you sleep for 8 hours, so we are estimating about half as many swallows as when you are awake for 240 swallows, to make a total of approximately 2,000 swallows per day.

If you are in the habit of swallowing incorrectly, that means you are doing the following:

- Pushing your tongue against your teeth approximately 2,000 times a day, which exerts more pressure than you might think. Wilson estimates the tongue presses the teeth with about four pounds of pressure and says it can lead to an abnormal bite and possibly orthodontic problems. Smart orthodontists will want to direct their patients to a speech-language pathologist trained in tongue thrust and swallowing or to a book like this to help them replace their hurtful habits with healthy ones. Because, even if they fix your teeth with braces, if you haven't corrected your bad oral habits, like a tongue thrust, the same issues will likely come back after your braces are taken off, unless you replace your hurtful habits with healthy ones. Perhaps this is why many orthodontists now ask you to wear your retainers for life.

- Pushing your tongue against your teeth also pulls on your jaw joints and ligaments over 2,000 times a day, a situation that can force the lips and facial muscles to contract to keep your tongue from sticking out of your mouth.

- Clenching your teeth down hard when you swallow over 2,000 times a day puts unnecessary wear and tear on your teeth and your jaw joints. Lighter touching is okay; however, excessive pressure creates undue wear on the joint structures.

- Tightening your neck muscles every time you swallow means that 2,000 times per day you needlessly tighten muscles that may already be overworked and strained. This tightening process can compress the structures in your neck. I have had some patients who were surprised that their neck pain could be reproduced every time they swallowed incorrectly.

The tongue and several important neck muscles attach to the hyoid bone, a small horseshoe-shaped bone just above the trachea (see Figure 6.2 on page 87). Keeping your tongue anchored on the roof of your mouth helps keep these structures stabilized while you swallow. The following exercise demonstrates how important good posture is for healthy swallowing. Then you will assess how you typically swallow.

EXERCISE \ *Swallowing with Poor Posture*

With a small amount of water in your mouth, look up at the ceiling and try to swallow. Is it easy or difficult to swallow in this posture? What happens to the position of your tongue and teeth?

While doing this exercise, I suspect you discovered that not only was it difficult to swallow with your head so extended but also your teeth probably had to clench together fairly hard in order for you to swallow the water. This exercise uses an exaggerated posture, but any poor posture can create havoc with your swallowing. Table 6.1 on the next page compares what happens during normal swallowing to what happens when swallowing with a tongue thrust.

Just as poor posture and cervical-spine problems set the stage for poor swallowing habits, your tongue's position can affect cervical and neck function. This is part of the reason toning and training your tongue and learning to swallow correctly are often so important for people suffering from neck pain and headaches. The structures of your head, neck, and jaw are all interrelated. You can't treat one without affecting the other connected parts.

How Do You Swallow?

At the beginning of this chapter, you tried to assess how you typically hold your tongue. Now try to see how you actually swallow. I say, "try," because whenever you start to think about something you do subconsciously, it can feel awkward or even forced. Sometimes it is hard to get an accurate picture the first time. So check occasionally over the next couple of days to see how you swallow when you aren't thinking about it.

Right now, you can get something to drink (preferably water) so you can practice swallowing while reading the rest of this chapter. If you can't get a drink right now, you can practice swallowing your saliva. It will help if you have a mirror to observe yourself in and a pencil and sheet of paper so you can write down the results as you go.

If you have a drink, you will be able to perform this assessment more quickly. If you are using your saliva, you will have to wait until enough collects each time to practice swallowing. You will swallow three to four times to assess each area, paying attention to different aspects of the swallowing process. It will help you to remember if you write down your answers after each trial.

1. Swallow and notice what happens to your **tongue**.
    - Does the tip of your tongue touch your front teeth at any time when you swallow?

- What does the middle of your tongue do as you swallow?

2. Swallow and notice what happens to your **teeth.**
   - Do your teeth touch at anytime during the swallowing process?
   - If your teeth touch, does it involve your front or back teeth or both?
   - Do they momentarily touch lightly or do they clench down firmly?

3. Place your hand around the back of your neck, swallow, and notice what happens to the **muscles below the base of your skull.**
   - Can you feel any of these muscles contract?

4. Swallow and notice what happens to your **lips and/or mouth.**
   - Did your lips noticeably move?

5. Swallow and notice what happens to your posture.
   - Does your head move when you swallow?

Table 6.1: Normal Swallow and Tongue-Thrust Swallow[17]

NORMAL SWALLOWING	SWALLOWING WITH A TONGUE THRUST
Tip of tongue goes to the ridges and segmentally presses the food or liquid along the roof of the mouth to the back of the throat. The tip of the tongue does not touch the front teeth.	Tip of the tongue typically pushes forward against the front or bottom teeth or between them at some point in the swallow.
Generally, back teeth touch lightly, if at all, when you are in good posture and using normal tongue function.	Teeth may touch firmly when swallowing, especially if you are in poor posture.
Very little, if any, contraction of the neck muscles at the base of the skull.	Muscle contractions and activity in the muscles at the base of the skull.
No head movement.	Head extension or forward craning.
No extra lip activity.	Lip activity is common.

What You Can Do to Swallow Correctly

You should practice swallowing correctly, especially if any of the following occurred while you were assessing your current swallowing habits:

- Your tongue tip touched the front of your top or bottom teeth at any point during swallowing.

- Your teeth were touching lightly before swallowing or they clenched together firmly during swallowing.

- Your head and lips noticeably moved or the neck muscles at the base of your skull contracted when you swallowed.

To practice swallowing correctly, I suggest using the series of steps based on those described by TMJ expert Steven Kraus.[18] He breaks down the steps involved in swallowing liquids, but you can apply the same principles when you swallow food. After reading these steps through, practice swallowing several times. Remember, good posture is important when you are swallowing, so sit up tall as you experiment with these steps.

1. Your tongue should already be resting along the roof of your mouth on "the spot," as we discussed earlier in this chapter. You need to make your tongue rest in the correct position regularly to swallow correctly.

2. When you place a cup to your mouth, your tongue should not push against the cup.

3. As water enters your mouth, let your tongue drop down to collect the liquid.

4. Swallowing starts when you close your lips and the tip of your tongue goes back to its resting position, or "the spot," and helps stabilize the lower jaw. That is where a wave of the tongue starts on the alveolar ridge, where those bumps or ridges give your tongue some traction to push off and initiate the swallow.

5. Next, your tongue segmentally squeezes and waves the fluid or food along the roof of your mouth from front to back toward the

back of your mouth and your swallowing tube (esophagus), like a peristaltic wave.

6. Your top back teeth should touch lightly on your bottom teeth. This helps stabilize the lower jaw as well. However, since the purpose is to ease the pressure on the joints, it is important to note that many people's teeth do not touch at all when they swallow, and this is fine, as long as the rest of the process is correct.

7. Your tongue then returns to anchor in its postural resting position on the roof of your mouth, allowing your head, neck, and jaw to relax.

8. Your head and neck muscles and lips should not noticeably move or contract when you swallow.

Swallowing food occurs in much the same way as swallowing liquid. In this case, however, the tongue has to gather the food and squeeze it along the roof of the mouth to the swallowing tube, which leads to the stomach. It does this in much the same way as toothpaste is squeezed out of its tube.[19] Chewing should typically occur on both sides of your back teeth simultaneously.[20]

Remember, people with TMJ disorders frequently have weak areas in their tongue. Tongue thrusters tend to use a mash-and-swallow technique instead of a segmental front-to-back wave-swallowing technique. This is why the tongue exercises in this chapter are so important. You must tone and retrain your entire tongue so it can do its job correctly.

The Development of Swallowing Habits

A healthy, mature swallow develops slowly. Babies have an infantile swallow and keep their tongue on the floor of their mouth. During this stage, breast-feeding or the use of an appropriate nipple can prevent the early development of hurtful swallowing habits.

When the child begins to stand upright and walk, as early as twelve to fifteen months of age, a mature swallow starts to develop. If your child has a displaced tongue, cannot seal his or her lips, or breathes through his or her mouth, your child's swallow will probably not develop correctly. As many as 80 percent of children who swallow incorrectly have problems with their bite, which can eventually lead to TMJ-related problems.[21]

Some common childhood behaviors that can cause problems, and suggestions about how to avoid them, are discussed below. Parents and health-care workers who treat children should help them learn healthy habits and postures early in life.

Common Childhood Behaviors that May Lead to Problems, and Healthy Alternatives

While nursing is what nature intended from the standpoint of encouraging normal development of the tongue and swallowing, it is not always an option. Bottles and pacifiers are often used instead. Often, these nipples are not shaped naturally or are used for too long and can lead to the development of an abnormal swallow and tongue position. Here are some recommendations, including those of Hilary Wilson, a speech-language pathologist who is specially trained in swallowing disorders and tongue thrust.[22]

- If pacifiers or bottles are used, be sure to use an ergonomic type nipple like the NUK brand that simulates the shape that a real nipple would assume during nursing.[23] Sippee cups and even sports bottle tops can also be problematic. Try using a cup with a straw instead. A child's lips need to be able to maintain closure, but the lips are not fully closed when the child has a pacifier or thumb in his or her mouth. If the lips are partially separated this way for long periods, it can lead to problems like a short upper lip.

- Thumb sucking and other hurtful oral habits should be discouraged because they can adversely affect the normal growth and development of the structures of the mouth and usually result in problematic tongue and swallowing habits. Thumb sucking can change the shape and development of the hard palate, usually making it too tall. Eventually, these hurtful oral habits can predispose a child to TMJ-related problems. Wilson recommends you discontinue the use of bottles, pacifiers, and sippee cups after age two or when teeth come in.

- For normal oral facial development, including healthy swallowing, the child needs to breathe through the nose. Work to resolve any airway obstructions that prevent your child's ability to breathe through the nose, including allergies, enlarged tonsils, nasal obstructions, and deviated septums to name a few of the issues that can make the child into a mouth breather.

- Educate yourself, your children, and those you care for in the healthy habits discussed in this book and address any problems you encounter along the way to ensure you can be successful.

Carl: The No-No Example
Carl drinks six cans of cola a day. Carl has crooked posture and is often slouching or crossing his legs. Every time Carl swallows, his tongue pushes against his teeth and his lips and neck muscles contract. Unbeknownst to Carl, the caffeine from his cola makes his muscles more irritable and sore, sometimes triggering headaches. He pours his caffeinated drinks into cups full of ice. Carl drinks from a cup, and every time he takes a sip, he bends backward, which hyperextends his neck, and over time this action irritates his cervical spine and the muscles in his neck. When Carl finishes a drink he chews on the leftover ice, adding further stress to his jaw joint, and the cold ice irritates the already sore muscles in his mouth.

Wanda: The Yes-Yes Example
Wanda keeps a cup of water with a straw by her side to use to stay hydrated during the day. Her water is not so cold that her muscles are stressed by the intense chill that cold can sometimes cause. Wanda has good posture. Her tongue rests on "the spot" on the roof of her mouth, never touching her front teeth. When Wanda drinks, her tongue waves the water back, never touching her teeth. Her neck muscles and lips stay relaxed when she swallows. She never chews her ice. Wanda is healthy, hydrated, and a super swallower, to boot.

Swallowing Awareness and Retraining Exercises
Now that you better understand that swallowing is a very complex activity, you can use this increased awareness to improve the qual-

ity of your swallow. And yet you swallow all the time, even at night, without giving it much thought. This makes incorrect swallowing a hard habit to change. Remember, swallowing incorrectly can add strain to your jaw and related structures over a thousand times a day. If you have swallowed incorrectly for years, it may take weeks or months to permanently change your hurtful swallowing habit to a healthy one, but it is worth it.

Listed here are exercises and ideas to help you remember and reinforce the habit of swallowing correctly. Practice daily until you habitually swallow correctly. Check yourself weekly, then monthly, and then as needed to ensure you maintain your healthy swallowing habit. As you do the exercises, keep in mind the following tips:

- Your tongue should not press against the cup when you are drinking or your front teeth when you are swallowing.

- Swallowing is the only time your teeth come together. However, lightly—if at all—is better for worn-down jaw joints.

- Your head should not need to move and the neck muscles at the base of your skull should not have to contract for you to swallow.

- You should have no excessive lip movement when you swallow. If your lips purse, it sends a signal for your tongue to come forward to push off your lips rather than pushing off the alveolar ridge on the roof of your mouth.

- If you have difficulty sealing your lips because you have a short upper lip, it should be addressed as well, since this can make it more difficult to swallow correctly.

> EXERCISE \ *A Daily Drink and a Sign*
>
> For the next couple of weeks, you should keep a drink close by so you can practice swallowing correctly throughout the day. This will help keep you hydrated and give you opportunities to replace a hurtful habit. You can also make a sign to keep on the kitchen table or wherever you eat to remind you to swallow correctly.

This conscious training of swallowing should lead you to swallow correctly without even thinking about it—even in your sleep.

EXERCISE *"I Will Swallow Right All Night"*

Take a paper cup and write on it with a marker: "Swallow Correctly!" After brushing and rinsing your teeth before you go to bed, take a few swallows of water correctly. Then say aloud three times: "I will swallow right all night." This helps reinforce the correct way to swallow. You will continue to swallow saliva all night subconsciously. Your goal is to program your mind to increase your awareness of this subconscious activity. Remember it is vital to have the correct sleeping posture to avoid a forward head position, which can cause you to clench, thrust your tongue, and swallow incorrectly. You can also begin the day swallowing correctly by repeating this exercise first thing in the morning when you brush your teeth.

EXERCISE *Swallowing Food at Mealtime with a Mirror*

Chew a cracker or whatever you are eating for dinner. The chewing should take place in the molar region of your mouth. The *bolus*—that is, the soft lump of food—should be collected on the middle of your tongue. You then squeeze and wave the food along the palate to the back of the throat. Following the swallow, the tongue should be clean except for a few crumbs. Remember there should be no facial movement when swallowing, so you may need a mirror to check.[24]

On an interesting side note, W. R. Proffit, B. B. Chastain, and L. A. Norton showed that just like people can be right or left handed, they can be right or left tongued.[25] However, always chewing or swallowing on the same side can create an imbalance, so you may want to try to chew and swallow as evenly as you can.

Still Having Trouble?

If you use all the retraining methods mentioned in this chapter and are still having trouble positioning your jaw and swallowing correctly, you may need more help. If you cannot achieve the correct posture, reread the posture sections and try the postural stretches and exercises in Chapter 4. If you still can't achieve good posture, check with your doctor and have a physical therapist help you regain your cervical mobility and strength to get there. If you have good posture and you cannot get your tongue to work properly, work on your tongue toning and training.

If you are still not making progress, you may want to be assessed by a professional. Swallowing is a difficult habit to relearn, and you may need a speech-language pathologist who is specifically trained in tongue thrust and swallowing disorders to help you. Professionals have dedicated their lives to helping people to retrain their tongue and to swallow correctly, and we have just covered the tip of the proverbial iceberg. Speech-language pathologists specifically trained in tongue thrust and swallowing disorders report it can take up to six months to make behavioral changes permanent. But don't be discouraged, I often see some improvements in as little as a week or two.

Summary

Now that you know where your tongue should rest and how to tone and train it to be a lean, mean swallowing machine, let's review the primary goals of this chapter:

1. Hopefully, you are beginning to see how interrelated each of the PoTSB TLC steps are.

2. Your tongue needs to be able to rest and stay anchored on the roof of your mouth to initiate relaxation of the muscles and facilitate healthy breathing through your nose and diaphragm.

3. When speaking English, the tip of your tongue should only touch your front teeth when you say "th," as in the word *Thursday*. Otherwise, it should be gently suctioned on the roof of your mouth.

4. There are many hurtful habits, especially as children, that can adversely alter the development of normal swallowing, tongue position, and facial development.

5. You swallow more than two thousand times a day. It is important to swallow correctly, with the tongue pushing the food or fluid from the front to the back of the roof of the mouth.

6. Make yourself a checklist for change. Use Table 6.2 as an example.

Table 6.2: Checklist for Change: Tongue Training and Swallowing Correctly

HURTFUL HABIT	HEALTHY HABIT	CHECKLIST FOR CHANGE
My tongue rests against my teeth.	My tongue rests on "the spot" on the roof of my mouth.	I will do tongue push-ups, using five to ten Cheerios in the morning and at night. I will tone and train my tongue by clucking when I drive. I will set daily hourly alarm to do PoTSB TLC and ensure tongue is in correct position.
In speech, my tongue pushes against my front teeth when I say the letters L and S.	The tip of my tongue should only touch front teeth when I say "th."	I will practice the speech exercises in Chapter 6. I will schedule an appointment with a speech-language pathologist if I continue to need help.
My tongue pushes against my teeth when swallowing.	My tongue pushes off the alveolar ridge when swallowing and waves food or fluid backward.	I will practice swallowing with cup of water and straw during the day. I will practice saying "buttercup" rhythmically and succinctly. I will put sign and mirror on table to practice swallowing at meals. I will label paper cup "Swallow Correctly" and set it by sink to practice when brushing teeth in the morning and evening.

7

Step 5: Breathe Well

You may have been breathing since birth, but that doesn't mean you can't learn to breathe better. In this chapter, we look at the **B** in PoTSB TLC, which stands for "breathe well." Breathing properly is essential for healing a TMJ disorder, as well as for your overall health.

When we breathe, we inhale oxygen and exhale carbon dioxide gas. Oxygen is usually the focus since it is a primary source of energy. You already know that if you don't get oxygen, you will die. After just three to four minutes without oxygen, your brain cells will start to die. Chronically starving yourself of vital oxygen by not breathing correctly won't have the same dramatic effect—that is, it won't kill you in three to four minutes. However, if you breathe shallowly, quickly, and incorrectly, you may suffer the consequences of these important gases being imbalanced in a variety of ways, including aggravation of chronic TMJ-related disorders.

Running Out of Gas

Having the right balance and amount of the gases oxygen and carbon dioxide is critical for your body to work correctly. Oxygen shortage in the human body has been linked to every major illness category, including depression, anxiety disorders, migraine, heart disease, respiratory disorders, and digestive diseases.[1] Robert Fried's research associated diabetes with poor breathing characterized by short, irregular breaths, also known as hyperventilation syndrome.[2]

Just about any illness can be made worse by an imbalance of oxygen and carbon dioxide gases. Research has shown that decreased oxygen to part of the brain seems to be intimately linked to migraine headaches.[3] It has also been shown that inhaling pure oxygen for 5 to 15 minutes can ease the pain of cluster-type headaches.[4] On the other hand, breathing too rapidly can actually cause you to get rid of too much carbon dioxide.

Chronic overbreathing can cause CO_2 levels in the blood to drop by 50 percent. Although we are often told that carbon dioxide gas is "waste," it plays a critical role in many bodily functions. Running too low on this important gas can wreak havoc with the pH balance in your blood.[5] This chemical change results in your sensory and motor nerves becoming more irritable—all because of low CO_2.[6] This means low CO_2 could make your sensory nerves more sensitive to irritants, which could, in turn, make you feel more pain than normal. And perhaps if your motor nerves become more jittery it might make you more likely to clench and grind your teeth or tense your muscles. New research links hyperirritable nerves with a multitude of chronic pain conditions, including TMJ disorders. These connections should be researched. Perhaps learning to breathe more slowly and regularly could normalize the CO_2 levels and, in turn, calm the nerves, making them less irritable without the use of drugs or surgery…just plain, old healthy breathing.

Your breathing is affected by many factors, including temperature, pain, fear, excitement, and happiness. It can also be influenced for good or bad by your fitness level. Healthy high-performance athletes and those who exercise regularly strengthen their breathing muscles and improve their body's ability to gather and use oxygen and get rid of the right amount of carbon dioxide.

Chest Breathing Is Breathing Turned Upside Down

Normal breathing should be slow, effortless, and rhythmic, drawn through your nose and using your diaphragm. Your diaphragm is a muscle that attaches below your lungs and to your ribs. It allows your

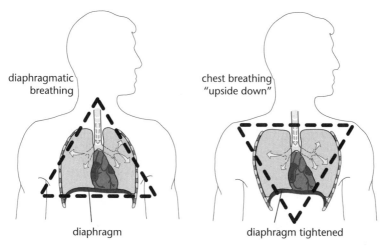

diaphragmatic breathing

chest breathing "upside down"

diaphragm

diaphragm tightened

FIGURE 7.1: Diaphragmatic breathing versus chest breathing

lungs to fully expand downward and outward. If you imagine a triangle with your head on top of the point and your diaphragm along the wide base, the bottom of the triangle should expand when you breathe in (see Figure 7.1). However, most of the patients I see are chest breathers who breathe too fast and only partially expand their diaphragm. It is as if their breathing triangle is turned upside down. With the diaphragm tight, the lungs have to inefficiently expand upward into the chest instead of downward (see Figure 7.1). This requires the neck muscles to lift the chest to make room for the lungs to expand on top and is also called *apical*, reverse, or upper thoracic chest breathing. When sitting quietly, you should breathe about 12 to 15 breaths per minute.[7] Chest breathing is tense, more shallow, and not as efficient as relaxed diaphragmatic belly breathing, so you must breathe more rapidly to compensate for the diaphragm not fully expanding. It is as if you are trying to fill your lungs with a one-third cup instead of a larger one cup, taking three times more effort. This can cause some people to hyperventilate. Because the neck muscles must contract frequently and lift your rib cage to help you breathe, this can lead to irritation and dysfunction in the muscles that connect to your head, neck, and jaw, which are not designed to be your primary breathing muscles. Instead, your diaphragm should be your primary breathing muscle. Dr. Fried says this "partial contraction of the diaphragm is part of the pattern of muscle tension in a stress response." So basically, stress partially tightens your diaphragm so it can't fully expand, which results in your neck muscles lifting your chest to compensate so your lungs have somewhere to expand and fill with air.[8]

The Obstacles to Breathing Your Best

So why are we not breathing correctly? The following factors are some of the most common obstacles to healthy breathing.

Stress

We just discussed the role stress plays in tightening your diaphragm so that it can't fully expand. How does stress do this? There is much still to learn, but we know that stress triggers the sympathetic nervous system's fight-or-flight response. It is called fight-or-flight because it harkens back to the response animals make under stress: They typically fight back or take flight and run away (see Chapter 11). Quick, shallow breaths are characteristic of this stress response. Have you ever noticed how your breathing is quick and shallow when you are stressed? People who are often anxious, stressed work-a-holics, or those who want everything to be perfect tend to overbreathe. The technique of breathing slowly through your nose and using your diaphragm has been taught throughout history to promote relaxation and health and is one of the best ways to switch gears from the fight-or-flight response to the more calming rest-and-digest mode.

Hyperventilation: Breathing Too Fast

Hyperventilation occurs when you overbreathe beyond what your body actually needs—often more than 15 to 20 breaths per minute, and it may become as high as 30 breaths per minute during a particularly stressful situation. Actually, breathing erratically and hyperventilating, or overbreathing, is a normal reaction to stress.[9] This may happen when your heartthrob walks into the room or you crash into the car in front of you when driving. The problem lies when we chronically overbreathe or breathe erratically. Perhaps we forget to normalize our breathing once the stressful event ends, or we constantly feel stressed or anxious and thus constantly tend to over-breathe.

Hypoventilation: Breathing Too Slow

Hypoventilation is less common, and it occurs when you don't breathe enough. According to the National Institutes of Health, obesity is the most common cause of hypoventilation. The excess weight applies pressure on the person's chest, making it difficult to breathe, and usually results in the body having too much carbon dioxide and too little oxygen. Clinically, I notice that my larger patients tend to be uncomfortable lying flat on their back and may have to sleep on their sides. Many suffer from sleep apnea as well.[10]

Mouth Breathing

Mouth breathers must keep their lips apart and their tongue can't rest on the roof of their mouth, because their tongue blocks the air from coming in and out of their mouths. All of this makes it difficult to breathe using the diaphragm, and their neck muscles kick in to compensate. Whenever I have a cold and am forced to breathe through my mouth, I am miserable. My mouth gets dry, my lips get chapped, and my head and neck hurt (partly because the accessory breathing muscles in my neck work overtime lifting my chest). I also have trouble sleeping and usually get a headache. Unfortunately, for some people, this is a way of life, even when they don't have a cold. However, it does not need to be that way. If your nasal passages are obstructed, talk to your physician and get help to open them up. Enlarged tonsils, a deviated septum, and asthma are some of the other problems that can adversely affect the way you breathe.

Maria: A Mouth Breather

I recently had an early adolescent in my class named Maria. She had already worn out 50 percent of the ball, or condyle, of her jaw joint. One of her primary problems was that she had never been able to breathe through her nose. She had a nasal obstruction that forced her to breathe through her mouth since she was a child. That created a cascade of hurtful habits. In order to breathe through her mouth, she brought her head forward and had to take her tongue off "the spot," to allow the air to pass through her mouth. With her tongue thrust against her teeth, she did not swallow or speak correctly, and this lack of tongue pressure on the roof of her mouth meant her lower jaw and face developed differently. Her upper lip was tight because she had to keep her mouth open to breathe. All this damage was caused so she could breathe through her mouth. While mouth breathing was by no means the only contributing factor to the wear and tear on her jaw joint, it was certainly a significant contributor. It would help if dentists and doctors had taught her these principles or could have helped her parents realize early on the consequences of mouth breathing and made appropriate steps to open her airway and learn healthy habits before most of her development occurred.[11]

Poor Posture

A slouched-forward head posture, with your shoulders rounded, scrunches your chest and abdominal cavity, making it difficult to breathe correctly. So healthy posture will help you breathe better. As you elevate your head and shoulders you open your chest, allowing more room for your lungs and diaphragm to do their jobs. Good posture also sets the stage for you to breathe through your nose, close your lips, and keep your tongue on the roof of your mouth, actions which are essential to healthy breathing.

Vanity

Thank goodness corsets are no longer in style, but trying too hard to pull in your belly and keep it flat makes it very hard for the diaphragm to do its job. Tight clothes that squeeze your abdomen will make it harder for you to breathe. Therefore, it is time to get rid of that girdle and those tight jeans and start breathing for a change.

Occupational Hazards

Certain occupational hazards tend to encourage mouth breathing. For example, wearing a surgical-type face mask can predispose you to mouth breathing.[12] Take note of your activities. If certain jobs force you to breathe through your mouth for long periods, see if there is a way to make modifications that allow nasal-diaphragmatic breathing. Stress may be the biggest occupational hazard of all.

Assess How You Breathe

Before we go further, let's assess how you actually breathe. It won't help you if you cheat, so answer honestly.

- Do you breathe through your mouth?
- Are your lips generally open?
- Are your lips dry or chapped?

If you answered yes to any of these questions, you are probably breathing incorrectly. Here is a more specific test you can use to assess the quality of your breathing.

EXERCISE \ **Breath Self-Test**

Begin by breathing the way you normally do. When you are ready, place one hand on your upper chest over your heart and the other hand on your abdomen over your belly button, as in Figure 7.2 on page 115. As you breathe, pay attention to which hand moves more. If the hand on your belly moves more, your breathing is likely diaphragmatic and healthy. If the hand on your chest moves upward, more or equally with your belly, or if your breathing is shallow, you can benefit from some improvement, which we will discuss later in this chapter.

EXERCISE \ **How Quickly Are You Breathing?**

To count your breaths per minute, look at a digital watch, sit in front of an analog clock with a second hand, or set a timer for one minute. Then count how many times you breathe in during that minute. If you are in a hurry, you can count your breaths during 15 seconds and multiply that number by four. It is a bit rough but takes less time.

Just by paying attention to your breathing rate, you can slow it down and in turn help switch gears from a stressful fight-or-flight mode to a calmer rest-and-digest state of being. Remember that your breathing muscles can get out of shape just like your other muscles. So start the exercises discussed later in this chapter slow and easy and increase only as tolerated. You should not feel dizzy or have discomfort. As always, check with your doctor if you have any concerns.

Slow and Steady Wins the Race

It is important to learn to calm your breathing so it is slow and rhythmic. There is no contest in which the person who takes the most breaths wins, and there is no prize for the person who breathes the quickest. Usually fast breaths are shallow upside-down breaths, and slow breaths tend to be relaxed, rhythmic, and diaphragmatic, making sure you don't run out of gas.

According to Fried, the average male breathes about 12 to 14 breaths per minute and the average female 14 to 16 breathes per minute. However, whatever your current breathing rate, most people can probably afford to slow it down a little bit. When people feel anxious, they easily breathe 20-plus breaths per minute. I recently clocked one patient's respiration veering out of control at 30 breaths per minute. At one point, I was feeling stressed by my book deadlines and timed my breathing rate at 20 breaths per minute, but after lying down for one minute, mentally applying the brakes, and switching gears to slow steady diaphragmatic breaths, I was comfortable and relaxed, taking only six breaths per minute. Once I resumed my activities, I was back to 12 to 14 breaths per minute. But taking a minute to relax and slow my breathing helped me feel more calm and in control. Some researchers link fast breathing or hyperventilation with anxiety, depression, panic attacks, and perfectionism.[13] Learning to switch gears and breathe slowly and effortlessly can help improve your heart function and lower your stress and anxiety levels, which can have a positive impact on TMJ disorders. (More information on stress is presented in Chapter 11.) Even the foods you eat can impact your breathing and stress level. Dairy products are common culprits and can cause excess mucus production, which in turn affects breathing. Also, high amounts of tyramine, which is present in varying amounts in most foods and increases as the food ages, is a common cause of food allergies and can lead to headaches and problematic breathing. This is one of the many reasons fresh foods are best.[14] (For more on headaches and food allergies see Chapter 10.)

What You Can Do to Breathe Well

Breathing experts agree that breathing correctly does more than just supply needed oxygen to weary bodies. It can calm frayed nerves and improve your emotional outlook on life, among many other psychological and emotional benefits. In fact, some yoga masters believe if you can control the breath, you can control the mind.[15] British researcher and physiotherapist Elizabeth Holloway published a landmark study involving 85 patients suffering from asthma. Half were given their usual asthma medications, while the other half were taught what she called the Papworth breathing method, based on the work of chest physician Dr. Claude Lum and physiotherapists Diana Innocenti and Rosemary Cluff at Papworth Hospital in Cambridge. At six and twelve month checks, those who had been taught to improve their breathing were able to breathe more slowly and had fewer asthmatic symptoms.[16] The breathing method was so successful that in one study 70 percent of their 320 patients were symptom free with 25 percent having only minor symptoms after treatment. I have tried to incorporate their primary methods throughout this chapter by making you aware of your breathing pattern and problems; educating you with the knowledge, exercises, and techniques needed so you can breathe slowly, rhythmically, and diaphragmatically; and finally by helping you learn to incorporate relaxation techniques at the first signs of stress.

Breathing is so subconscious that you breathe in and out about twelve to fifteen times a minute without ever thinking about it.[17] In the exercises that follow, you will practice becoming more conscious of your breathing. This doesn't mean you have to be aware of every breath, all day long, although you should periodically assess your breathing when you do your regular PoTSB TLC checks. Breathing well is the **B** in our acronym. By practicing some good breathing habits now, the time you spend breathing correctly can carry over into the breaths you take for the rest of your life.

Breathe with Your Diaphragm

Even though your diaphragm is your primary breathing muscle, you may not know where it is, how it works, or how to get it working at its best to improve your health. Your diaphragm is a parachute-shaped muscle that sits below your lungs and separates the upper chest cavity from your lower abdominal area. When you inhale, your diaphragm muscle contracts and pulls the parachute-shaped muscle down flat, as in Figure 7.1 on page 107. This allows your lungs to fully expand and fill to the brim with healthy, oxygen-laden air. The movement also massages the abdominal organs below, improving their function and ability to process and remove toxins. When your diaphragm relaxes, it floats back to its parachute shape, forcing air and waste out of your lungs as you exhale.

EXERCISE \ *Eight Steps to Proper Breathing*

Let's try some relaxed, rhythmic diaphragmatic breathing right now. Here are seven steps to guide you through the process. You can do these exercises sitting, standing, or lying down. However, lying down is often a more relaxing and ideal position to start with. Place one hand on your chest and one over your belly. It is a good idea to wear loose clothing or to loosen your belt and remove constrictions. Doing so will make it easier for you to breathe correctly.

1. **Start in good posture.** If you are sitting or standing, position your-self upright. If you are lying down, make sure you have your head supported in a balanced position, not too far forward.

2. Have your **tongue anchored on "the spot"** on the roof of your mouth.

3. Keep your **lips gently together** and slightly separate your teeth.

4. **Slowly inhale and exhale through your nose**, with your tongue on the roof of your mouth, teeth apart, and lips together. Breathing through your nose moisturizes and cleans the air and helps trigger your diaphragm to get to work. Your breathing rate should be calm and steady.

5. **Use your diaphragm,** not your chest. Your diaphragm is your primary breathing muscle, allowing the best lung "ventilation," and it should be doing most of the work, not your neck muscles. Put one hand on your chest and one hand on your belly to make sure the diaphragm is moving. If you are lying down, you can place your hand or a small book on your belly. The weight of the book or your hand gives you some feedback and something for your belly

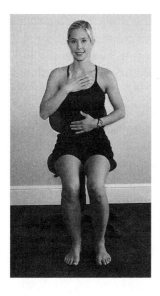

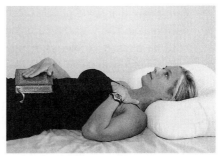

FIGURE 7.2: Diaphragmatic breathing while sitting or lying

to push against (see Figure 7.2). The book or hand on your belly should rise when you inhale or breathe in and fall when you exhale or breathe out. This is a great way to practice breathing first thing in the morning and just before bed.

6. Your **sides should expand** as you inhale, **as well as your belly.** Remember, your entire lower rib cage is expanding when you inhale. It may be tight, and it may take time to stretch back to normal.

7. Your **neck and shoulders should be relaxed**. Soften your neck, chest, and shoulders. Do not let your shoulders rise up toward your head as you inhale, which would indicate that you are still lifting your chest with your neck muscles to allow the lungs to expand upward like an upside down triangle instead of downward. This is a very common mistake and one most people are not even aware they are making. Let the tension in your belly, sides, and diaphragm melt away, allowing them to move in and out with the rhythmic tide of air flowing in and out of your body.

8. Your **breathing should be slow and steady**. Rhythmically count the seconds it takes to inhale and exhale. Continue to breathe slowly and rhythmically encouraging relaxation. If you are breathing too fast or irregularly, try to gently lengthen your breaths and make them more regular, as tolerated. Keep practicing until this rhythm feels comfortable and natural, but never stop breathing.

I am aware that some people breathe too slowly; however, since overbreathing is by far the most common problem, that is the focus I have taken. As always, remember that many factors affect your breathing, and you should be evaluated properly by a physician before starting any new exercise program.

This exercise works well right before going to bed. If you have had or are having a stressful day, it may help alleviate that stress as well. You can breathe in any position, but it often makes you feel more relaxed if you can find a safe place to lie down, even if it means shutting the door and lying on the floor. Whatever the position, you want to breathe comfortably through your nose and with your diaphragm. Now focus on relaxing, so you can help slow the acceleration and harmful consequences of unbridled stress.

Dr. Fried warns that doing too much too soon may make you feel light-headed, so start in a safe place, consciously using just a few slightly slower and more-relaxed breaths, and increase the depth and repetition as tolerated. As always, it is advisable to consult with your health-care provider before starting any new exercises or program.

EXERCISE \ *Stretch Your Diaphragm and Ribs*

A friend who is a talented opera singer introduced me to this next exercise, which is a variation of the one above. I thought I was a pretty good breather until I tried it. My belly moved but my sides were stiff. After a week of diligent practice, however, I had it down—and you can, too.

You can do this exercise, which helps stretch the diaphragm and ribs, in just about any position, but this is an easy one to practice when you are sitting in a boring class or meeting or waiting for an appointment. I will describe how to do the exercise in a sitting position.

Sitting with your hands on your knees in good posture, try breathing diaphragmatically. Make sure your abdominal area is free of restrictions. No tight pants, belts, or girdles are allowed. Your neck and shoulder muscles are relaxed, and you should feel your belly and ribs expand. Your tongue is on the roof of your mouth, teeth apart, and lips together. Make sure your shoulder and neck muscles are relaxed. As you breathe in and out through your nose, the bottom of your rib cage should expand fully to achieve a gentle stretch, which means your belly and your sides should expand, too. Often the ribs and diaphragm are tight from disuse due to chest breathing. Some people have difficulty getting any rib expansion. For others, it feels foreign and new, like driving a stick-shift car after years of driving an automatic. Eventually, your rib cage and diaphragm will fully expand, allowing you the mobility to breathe more calmly and efficiently. You can give yourself some feedback by straightening yourself and placing your hands on the sides of your lower ribs to help signal them to push outward against your hands as you breathe in.

As your ability to breathe consistently in a healthy way improves, you will be better able to maintain the right balance of oxygen and carbon dioxide in your body. Only do one or two repetitions, as very deep breathing can momentarily lower your blood CO_2 levels by 20 to 25 percent.[18] Once your ribs and diaphragm have stretched to normal length, these stretches can be discontinued, because your normal healthy breathing will maintain your new mobility.

EXERCISE \ *Skip and Slide*

This exercise can help those who breathe erratically to breathe more rhythmically. First, inhale, taking several short, rhythmic breaths. These are the "skips." Then, exhale in one long, even breath for the "slide." This exercise can help you steady and regulate your breathing. You can modify this exercise in several ways. You can reverse this process by inhaling in one long segment and exhaling in several short segments. Once you breathe rhythmically on a regular basis you can discontinue this exercise. You can use imagery to steady and slow your breathing, such as the ocean tide flowing in and out. You can even breathe to music. Find what works best for you.

EXERCISE \ *Count It Out*

If you are prone to overbreathe, you can slow it down by simply timing your breaths. Count the seconds it takes to inhale and exhale. You can slow your breaths by holding your breath one second longer after exhaling. When that pace is comfortable, you can add another second. You should stay in your comfort range where you are free from symptoms, not gasping for breath. If you are breathing in and out every two seconds, it means you are breathing thirty times every minute, which is too fast. My husband is a runner and in good health, so while he was sleeping, I decided to time his breaths. He inhaled for two seconds and exhaled for two seconds, so he was taking a breath every four seconds in a perfectly smooth and effortless rhythm. That would put him at 15 breaths per minute.

EXERCISE \ *Contract, Relax*

Since stress affects your breathing, you need to learn to relax. One technique is to contract a muscle group and then completely let it relax and lay limp. You can do this with each muscle group, and it can help you feel the difference between a tense muscle and a relaxed one. This is one of many techniques that can help you relax when you feel the onset of stress and tension. Find a technique that works best for you and use it. It can help you slow and control your breaths and better control your life.

Seek Professional Help

If you have difficulty breathing, it is important to see a doctor who can rule out any serious medical concerns. If you cannot breathe through your nose, you may also need more help than is offered in this book. The problem may be with your sinuses, allergies, a deviated septum, enlarged tonsils, asthma, even food allergies or something else. In this case, you may need to see an allergist or ear, nose, and throat doctor or expert in this area. Seriously consider all your options with the realization that all aspects of breathing through your mouth can adversely affect the growth and development of the mouth and face. So resolving the obstruction and teaching a young child, or yourself, healthy habits before this growth and development occurs can have a profound and beneficial impact. You may suffer from chronic anxiety or emotional tension that needs professional help to resolve. Assess and take care of both your mind and body.

Summary

If you are reading this book, then you are obviously breathing. While you likely seldom think about breathing and it doesn't seem that complicated, learning to breathe correctly can have a positive impact on your overall health, as well as that of your head, neck, and jaw. Let's review the main points:

1. Adequate levels of the gases oxygen and carbon dioxide are critical to your overall health and well-being.

2. Mouth breathing and quick shallow chest breathing are often a result of stress and anxiety, and can irritate neck muscles and aggravate headaches and TMJ-related disorders.

3. Good posture and breathing through your nose and diaphragm are essential for you to breathe properly.

4. Keeping your tongue on "the spot" and lips together forces you to breathe through your nose and can help trigger your diaphragm to do its job.

5. Make a plan to improve your breathing habits, which can include general exercise, the exercises in this chapter, stress management, and a diet of fresh, healthy foods.

6. Make yourself a checklist for change. Use the sample in Table 7.1 as a guide.

Table 7.1: Checklist for Change: Breathing Correctly

HURTFUL HABIT	HEALTHY HABIT	CHECKLIST FOR CHANGE
I breathe through my mouth and keep my lips apart.	I breathe through my nose and keep my lips closed.	To breathe at my best: I will check my PoTSB TLC hourly. I will stretch and train my short upper lip so I can keep my lips sealed. I will see a doctor if I can't get adequate air through my nose.
My current breaths per minute are 19 and they are short and shallow.	My goal is to breathe more diaphragmatically and calmly by decreasing my number of breaths per minute to 12.	I will hourly check my PoTSB TLC and time my breaths during the day. I will stretch my ribs and diaphragm with exercises when waiting for appointments. I will do cardiovascular exercise 3–5x/week for 30 minutes. I will practice slow, steady, effortless breathing every night for 5 minutes before bed.

8

Step 6: Care for Your Muscles

Did you know you have over 600 muscles in your body? In fact, when considered all together, muscles account for approximately 40 percent of the average person's body weight.

Every day we use and abuse our muscles, and too often we take them for granted. Perhaps because muscles cannot be seen on X rays, they are often overlooked as the cause of pain and dysfunction. Yet, our muscles cause us pain in more ways than you might imagine. A muscle spasm or imbalance can give you a headache, earache, or even a toothache. They can also change your bite, and cause and contribute to your joint clicking or locking. Muscles can be a major contributor to and cause of head, neck, and jaw pain. Tight, tense, and hyperactive muscles can put undue stress on the joint structures, causing the cartilage and disk to break down or tear or move these structures out of their proper place, thereby creating serious joint dysfunction.[1]

Malfunctioning muscles are especially common in people with TMJ-related disorders, including fibromyalgia and those who have experienced acute trauma such as a whiplash injury. In this chapter, we look at ways to care for our muscles and overcome muscle-related pain and dysfunction.

Myofascial Pain

Pain in the muscles of your head, neck, and jaw is one of the most common complaints from people who suffer from TMJ-related problems. We call this *myofascial* pain. *Myo* means "muscle." So what is *fascia*? Fascia is a connective tissue that runs through your body like netting. Your fascia holds and connects your muscles, organs, and body systems together. Therefore, although you might say you have "sore muscles" or "muscle pain," in the medical community we use the term *myofascial pain*.

The Pain Cycle

Injury, microtrauma, overuse, and abuse of your muscles can irritate and injure the muscles and associated soft tissue. As this tissue heals, it can shorten and tighten into a knot. This only causes further pain and does not allow the muscle to move or function properly. When your muscles are sore or painful, they become tighter. However, it takes more energy to keep a muscle tight. The muscle needs more food and oxygen to keep working, and working muscles also create more waste. If your muscles stay tense and tight, they can become weak and unhealthy.

This condition creates a cycle of pain and dysfunction. In a nutshell, the pain leads to muscle tension and guarding, which hinders circulation and makes the muscles tight. A tight muscle with poor circulation tends to become irritated and inflamed, which leads to

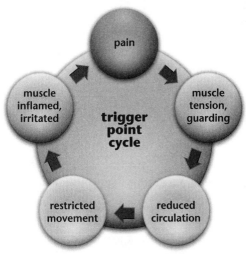

FIGURE 8.1: Muscle pain and tightness cycle[2]

more pain and dysfunction, and so on, until the cycle is broken (see Figure 8.1 on the previous page). So let's look at ways to break this vicious cycle.

To break the pain-tightness cycle, it is best to eliminate the irritants and "un-tighten" the muscles by releasing or undoing the knots and gently moving, elongating, and stretching the muscles.[3] This stretching must be done very carefully and over a period of time, because a sore muscle can be easily irritated. Usually, stretching feels great, but I recommend starting with only one or two new muscles a day, to see how you respond. Overstretching or stretching too hard can make the muscle more irritated instead of better. If you have fibromyalgia or health problems that may be a complication, you should check with your health-care provider before starting any exercise or stretching program. When in doubt, always check it out.

Myofascial Trigger Points

To understand myofascial pain, it is important to appreciate the interconnectedness of this system. Tightness in one myofascial area can pull, create stress, and adversely affect a distant area of the body. Believe it or not, scars, injuries, and tightness in the muscles and fascia as far away as the foot can adversely affect the posture of your head, neck, and jaw, because the parts of your body are all interconnected. Tight muscles can even squeeze and irritate nerves. Some people with irritated nerves often believe the problem is coming from their spine, when it might actually originate where the nerve is squeezed by a tight muscle.

A tight muscle in your jaw can adversely affect your bite and even cause a toothache in a healthy tooth. I have seen patients who have had root canals or teeth pulled to relieve a toothache. Much to their chagrin, these procedures didn't make their toothache go away, because the tooth was fine and the trigger point in a muscle was the real culprit. So please do not have an irreversible procedure when you can't specifically identify the cause. For example, if you have a sudden change in your bite, it could be the result of a muscle that is tight or in spasm. You don't want to rush out and have your bite altered, only to learn that the muscle spasm was temporary, but the bite change you rushed to have is permanent.

Dr. David Simons and the late Dr. Janet Travell, who was John F. Kennedy's physician in the White House, wrote *Myofascial Pain and Dysfunction: The Trigger Point Manuals,*[4] which are sometimes referred to as the "red bibles" because they seem to have the answers to most myofascial problems. Using medical lingo, they brilliantly describe in great detail almost every major muscle group in the body and explain not only pain patterns but also probable causes and treatments. They popularized the term *myofascial trigger points* as a result of their revolutionary efforts to understand and document myofascial pain, its causes, and treatments. Many of the concepts for this chapter are inspired by their work.

Trigger points are local areas of tenderness in a nodule of tight muscle, fascia, or tissue that triggers pain when pressed. Some trigger points feel like a knot or a taut rope. These tight bands can actually entrap nerves and blood vessels and disrupt the flow of the lymphatic system, which helps remove waste from your body.

You may be wondering how you find your trigger points. Since trigger points are spots on your body that trigger pain when pressed, you will find them as you press areas that are potentially problematic. However, keep in mind that trigger points can refer pain to other areas. For example, you can have an ache on the side of your head above your ear that is being triggered by a tight and tender muscle in the back of your neck. Even a toothache in a healthy tooth can be referred pain from a distant trigger point. Trigger points are most common in the postural muscles of the neck, shoulder, pelvic girdle, and the muscles used for chewing. Trigger points are generally classified into two categories: active and latent.

Active trigger points. If you have an active trigger point, you would probably be able to tell me where you are hurting without my even poking your muscles. It would refer pain at rest and/or when you press on or move the muscle. The muscle would be tight, tender, and weak.

Latent trigger points. Latent trigger points lurk in the shadows. They don't hurt until they are poked and prodded, and then you realize your muscle is sore. A latent trigger point is always tight and may also cause muscle weakness and dysfunction. A tight muscle cannot fully lengthen or obtain the nutrition it needs. Sedentary couch potatoes, or those who get little exercise, have a greater likelihood of developing latent trigger points.

The Causes of Muscle Pain and Trigger Points

The material in this section is largely based on clinical experience and the work of Gerwin;[5] *Simons, Travell, and Simons;*[6] *and Travell and Simons.*[7]

Travell and Simons say that treating the causes or perpetuating factors is the most important and yet most neglected part of the management of muscle pain. In *Myofascial Pain and Dysfunction,* they tell the story of a man who stepped in a hole in the sidewalk and broke his leg. He was treated and the bones in his leg healed, but a few months later, he stepped in the same hole and broke his leg again. No one had addressed the cause by patching the hole.[8] Similar to our earlier example, if you treat muscle pain without "patching the holes," then you are doomed to endless cycles of treatment and relapses.

If you have one leg that is shorter than the other, your body is unbalanced and stressed every time you are on your feet. If you sleep on your stomach every night, your head is probably extremely rotated and pushing hard against the bed or pillow, putting pressure on your jaw and neck the entire night, and side sleeping also rotates and presses on the weight-bearing head, shoulder, and hip. You may have gotten away with these hurtful habits until some event put you over the edge. Now, you are having trouble getting the pain to go away and wondering why. To achieve the best results, you need to address as many of these kinds of "holes," or hurtful habits, as you can, even if you have been accustomed to getting away with them. In the long run, you and your body will be happier.

The place to start is by understanding what has caused your trigger points to develop. Trigger points are typically activated or perpetuated by one of more of the following:

Acute overload or abuse (occurring over hours or days). This involves the sudden contraction or overstretching of the involved muscle, which can result from an auto accident, fall, blow to the face or head, lengthy dental procedure, sudden strain or pull, vomiting, or other similar event.

Chronic overuse (occurring over weeks, months, or years). Poor posture or body mechanics, overwork, hurtful habits and fatigue, and ongoing mechanical stresses such as a leg-length discrepancy or hemipelvis are some of the factors that predispose or perpetuate muscle pain and dysfunction. Spending lots of time on the computer or phone or lugging around a purse or briefcase are prime examples.

Keeping a muscle in a shortened position for a long time. This problem can occur from clenching your teeth or sleeping on your stomach, with your arm overhead or positioned by your face, or from just remaining in the same position for an extended period of time. Other common examples include studying in bed, sitting on a wallet all day, or watching TV at an angle with your head turned for hours.

Not getting enough good sleep. This is really important and may require the help of your doctor or a sleep specialist. You need the right quality and quantity of sleep to be healthy and to feel good.

Nutritional and metabolic deficiencies, disorders, or imbalances. A competent physician can rule out any of the following nutritional issues:[9]

- low levels of B-1, B-6, B-12, and folic acid; vitamin C deficiency; anemia; and lack of calcium, potassium, iron, magnesium, and several trace minerals essential for normal muscles
- thyroid dysfunction, hypoglycemia, and gout
- nicotine use, tobacco smoking, and excess caffeine intake, which make your muscles more irritable

Other trigger points. One trigger point can activate other trigger points in nearby muscles, called *satellite trigger points*. Unfortunately, this can progress to a chronic condition and include most of the muscles in your body.

Psychological factors. These factors include anxiety, tension, depression, and feelings of hopelessness. Negative emotions lead to more pain than positive emotions. We too often ignore our mental and emotional health. Our brain and emotions are as intricately tied to our bodies as are our legs and arms; however, we just don't always see the connections. Take the necessary steps to ensure that both aspects are given appropriate attention.

Pain from arthritic, inflamed, or dysfunctional joints that are located nearby. If your jaw is inflamed or neck joints are arthritic or dysfunctional, you will often have irritable painful muscles around those joints. Trigger points also tend to develop around pinched nerves.

Cold temperatures. Cold can activate trigger points in some people. This "chill stress" can be caused by air conditioning, drafts, cold weather, or even cold drinks. Chill stress is more common when you are tired or have thyroid dysfunction. My fibromyalgia patients are extremely sensitive to cold as well.

Viral illness. These illnesses include the herpes simplex type 1 virus that causes mouth, canker, and common cold sores.

Infections and allergic rhinitis. These infections can be bacterial or viral.

Visceral disease. For example, it is common knowledge that people with heart troubles often experience chest, shoulder, or arm pain.

Trigger Point Treatment

Trigger points need to be treated effectively to break the cycle of pain, spasm, and loss of function. Keep in mind that it will take both time and effort to improve and eliminate trigger points. Trigger point treatment should include:

- Identifying and eliminating the causes and perpetuators of the problems, which is the most overlooked step. This book is my attempt to help change that.

- Making sure you get the right amount of quality sleep for you. Studies have shown that poor quality and quantity of sleep will result in increased muscle pain.

- Regaining and maintaining the full range of motion of the muscle. This is essential. Treatment should continue until this goal has been achieved, and it may require the assistance of a physical therapist.

Trigger point treatments are performed by a trained therapist or specialist. However, you can learn to do some level of problem solving and healthy movement for yourself. Depending on the severity of your issue, the general stretches and exercises presented in this book will improve motion and provide relief. Because everyone and their situation is a little different, I always recommend seeing a professional who can modify the program specifically for you, but this section will give you lots of ideas.

Find and release the trigger point. You or a friend can feel for trigger points along your muscles and gently knead or release them. Be gentle and start with only one or two spots to determine how you tolerate the process. If you are hypersensitive, any pressure that is too strong can make you feel worse. So you be the judge for your own body.

You can even find and massage trigger points on the muscles inside of your mouth (see Table 8.1 on page 132). First, make sure you do not have long nails. Then, with clean hands or wearing surgical gloves, slide your forefinger and thumb along your cheek to feel for and treat trigger points. Either your thumb or forefinger will be inside your mouth, while the other finger helps with balance and counterpressure on the opposing side. Please take note of the direction in which the muscle fibers run in the illustrations for each muscle, as knowing this can improve the effectiveness of any release or massage-type techniques inside or outside of your mouth.

Trigger point pressure release is when you apply gentle pressure to help the trigger point to let go before stretching the muscle.[10] **I tell my patients it is like melting butter with your fingers.** I apply gentle pressure on the trigger point and it should be like that "feel-good" pressure you get when someone rubs your neck. Then I wait on top of the trigger point. You can imagine if you pressed a warm finger on a stick of cold butter and waited; eventually your warm finger will melt the butter and sink into the stick. In healthy muscles, this can happen too and it is really cool to feel a trigger point "melt" in your hands. I then treat other trigger points within that muscle and bring the person through his or her full available, normal range of motion. You can purchase a trigger point instrument to help treat those hard-to-reach spots, or you can make one with something as simple as a ball and a pair of pantyhose. To learn how to make a trigger point instrument or which ones our patients like best, go to my website at www.tmjhealingplan.com.

Massage techniques are multiple and instinctive. Many people with trigger points are seen rubbing their necks or massaging their temples. If I don't have the luxury of being treated by someone else, I first release my trigger points by applying pressure as we just discussed. Then, I may lubricate the skin before massaging, which helps to decrease friction, or I can even work the muscle through my clothes if I need to apply relief when I am in a place where I cannot work directly on the skin. Then I slowly stroke the muscle in the same direction as the tight muscle fibers in order to work out the "knots." I do this as gently as I possibly can while still obtaining the desired results. If I have the time and resources, I apply moist heat to the muscles for 5–10 minutes when I am done with my self-massage, and then I move to maintain motion. Remember, pressure can irritate some people, particularly those with fibromyalgia or those who are hypersensitive. To be most effective, you must have an understanding of the anatomy and direction of the fibers and know the appropriate level of pressure that should be applied. Later in this chapter, I will introduce some of the most problematic muscles involved in TMJ disorders, including anatomy, direction of the muscle fibers and common trigger points, and typical pain referral patterns. But remember, no two people are exactly the same.

More trigger point release techniques and modalities. There are a variety of ways to alleviate trigger points.[11] I will briefly touch on a few of the most common techniques. These should be provided by a physical therapist or health-care professional specifically trained in treating TMJ disorders and myofascial pain.

- *Spray and stretch* involves applying a cool, vaporous spray in sweeping motions along the fibers of the muscle, then passively (i.e., the therapist, not you, does all the work) stretching the muscle and following the treatment with moist heat. According to Simons, Travell, and Simons, spray and stretch is probably the single most effective way to inactivate an active new trigger point and regain motion.[12]

- Massage techniques such as strumming, friction, and ice massage.

- Myofascial release is a combination of hands-on techniques used to release restrictions in the muscle and fascia.
  Other modalities used by physical therapists include:

- Ultrasound with or without medications on the surface of your skin or the use of iontophoresis, a type of electric-current treatment, which can decrease inflammation and irritation and increase warmth and circulation.

- Various forms of electrical stimulation to help release trigger points and help break the cycle so muscles can heal. Intraoral probes can be used for trigger points inside the mouth.

- Manual techniques designed to calm the muscle and regain motion and function, including reciprocal inhibition, contract-relax, post-isometric relaxation, muscle energy techniques, and specific stretches and exercises tailored to your individual needs.[13]

- Trigger point injections are done by specially trained health-care providers who inject medicine such as an anesthetic into the trigger point to help the site become less irritated. Dry needling of the trigger point can also be helpful.

Common Muscle Myths
Travell and Simons point out four common misconceptions about myofascial pain, and I have added a fifth one that I am confident they would approve of.[14]

1. **It is all in your head.** Unfortunately, too many people in real pain have had someone say this to them. According to Drs. Travell and Simons, many physicians dismiss myofascial pain

because the X rays and lab findings are normal; therefore, it must be "in your head." However, more and more physicians are learning about trigger points.

2. **It will go away in its own.** Although active trigger points may spontaneously improve by becoming latent, they don't just "go away" on their own. These latent trigger points are ready to be activated by any trivial irritant. You need to identify and deactivate those latent trigger point time bombs.

3. **Don't take it seriously.** Myofascial pain can cause a sudden cramp in a muscle serious enough to cause accident, injury, and in some cases suicide. Myofascial back pain is one of the major causes of work-related disability.

4. **If your pain goes away, then everything is fine.** If you were my patient and complained of pain in your left arm and chest and it improved with stretching, I would still send you to the hospital for an evaluation to rule out cardiac distress.

5. **The movement myth.** Many people seem to think that if something hurts, you should immobilize it and let it rest. Although it is true that overloading and overworking a muscle can be detrimental, gentle, healthy movement is essential to healing. In fact, Travell and Simons say to ensure continued relief of trigger points, you should establish a home program of stretching and moving through your full normal range of motion.[15] Your muscles must move to maintain their health, length, and strength. My patients who move and exercise safely and regularly get better faster. Let me give you an example of the power of movement:

Cynthia: Reaching for the Top Shelf

One day, as I was straining to reach something on a top shelf, I pulled a muscle in my neck and shoulder area that became extremely painful. I could feel it start to spasm and tighten to protect itself from the strain. Most people I know would have reacted by trying to immobilize the area, thinking they were helping to protect their muscles by not moving them. If I had stopped moving, I could have ended up with several days or weeks of pain and discomfort. Luckily, as a physical therapist, I have some experience in this area. I immediately started moving the muscle with gentle shoulder shrugs and circles until I could feel it start to relax again. I did a few gentle stretches in the pain-free range to restore the muscle length, and took a few deep abdominal breaths. Then I found a step stool, reached my item without any strain, and went about my day with no residual symptoms.

Restore and Maintain a Full Range of Motion

For an impaired muscle to become healthy again, it needs to be able to move through its full normal range of motion. If you have gone to the effort of working on and releasing trigger points and want to get the best results, you will follow the treatment with gentle movements throughout the day. You must remember that there are 24 hours in a day. If you stretch and move the muscle for 30 minutes and then tighten and tense the muscle for 23½ hours, you will probably lose the battle. Gently move your muscles throughout the day, and identify and eliminate the causes of tightness and irritation.

However, keep in mind that if you have overly loose joints and connective tissue, you and anyone else who stretches you must be very careful to stop in your normal range and not stretch the muscle to your exaggerated available range. Many people with TMJ disorders are hypermobile, due to loose joints. You must be very careful not to stretch a muscle too far. It is better to understretch rather than overstretch. Also, keep in mind that if you have had tight, tense muscles for years, they won't change length in a day and could be injured if you try to make them do so. It is best to consult with a physical therapist.

Which Muscles Refer Pain Where?

To begin to work toward healthier muscles, you need to understand something about each of the muscle groups that are most frequently the culprits in head, neck, and jaw disorders. Table 8.1 on the next page lists key painful areas and the major muscle groups most often known for referring pain to each region. For each painful area,

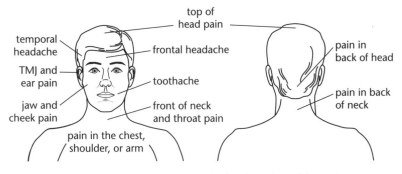

FIGURE 8.2: Common locations for head, neck, and jaw pain

Table 8.1: Head, Neck, and Jaw Pain and Common Muscle Culprits[16]

PAINFUL AREA	LIKELY MUSCLE CULPRITS	PAINFUL AREA	LIKELY MUSCLE CULPRITS
TMJ and ear pain	Lateral pterygoid Masseter Sternocleidomastoid Medial pterygoid	Toothache	Temporalis Masseter Digastric
Jaw and cheek pain	Sternocleidomastoid Masseter Lateral pterygoid Trapezius Digastric Medial pterygoid	Pain in the back of the neck	Trapezius Multifidi Splenius cervicis
		Pain in the front of the neck and throat	Sternocleidomastoid Digastric Medial pterygoid
Temporal headache, or pain on the side of the head	Trapezius Sternocleidomastoid Temporalis Splenius cervicis Suboccipital(s) Semispinalis capitis	Pain in the back of the head	Trapezius Sternocleidomastoid Semispinalis capitis and semispinalis cervicis Splenius cervicis Suboccipital(s) Digastric Temporalis
Frontal headache	Sternocleidomastoid Semispinalis capitis		
Pain on top of the head	Sternocleidomastoid Splenius capitis	Pain in the chest, shoulder, or arm	Pectoralis

the muscle most likely to be the culprit is listed first, followed by secondary culprits in the order of their probable correlation to the pain. I have only listed the muscles we discuss in this book. You must become a detective to identify the hurtful habits perpetuating your trigger points before you can eliminate them. When you understand the location, action, and pain referral patterns of each muscle, you can teach yourself gentle stretches to help restore length and function and decrease pain. You should check these muscles regularly by gently pressing each muscle with the flat part of your fingers, trying to detect tenderness or knots. In medical terms, this is called *palpation*. When you press, or palpate, you use your fingers to sense the condition of the muscle, or whatever structure you are trying to assess. By palpating in this manner, you can identify and eliminate latent trigger points before they become active. This type of awareness and healthy activity will save you some pain and problems now and down the road.

In the pages that follow, I explain the following five factors for each muscle group:

Location. I have listed and shown in illustrations the location of each muscle so you can more easily find it on your body.

Pain referral and symptoms. Pain referral relates to patterns in which trigger points in certain muscles have been commonly demonstrated to refer pain and symptoms within the muscle itself or to distant areas. This helps you, as the detective, determine if your symptoms could be linked to trigger points for this muscle. If, for example, you experience pain on the side of your head and toothaches, you can look at Table 8.1 and see that the temporalis muscle is the only one listed for both symptoms, which means this might be a good muscle for you to check first. You can also look at trigger-point and pain-referral pictures for each muscle in this chapter and see which ones correlate with your symptoms. Keep in mind that there are usually multiple muscles involved, including many, sometimes overlapping, referral patterns. Evaluation by a health-care professional is always recommended to rule out serious complications or causes for pain.

Action. The action explains the primary function of the muscle, which can help you better understand what might be causing problems and how you can reinforce or create healthy habits. Keep in mind that muscles can contract as they shorten and lengthen. I have primarily listed their shortening, or *concentric*, action, but you can usually reverse it and assume the muscle lengthens in the opposite direction. For example, the quadriceps muscles straighten the knee (e.g., when kicking a ball); however, the quadriceps also contract in a lengthening fashion to help lower or bend your leg as you walk down stairs. Lengthening contractions are called *eccentric* contractions and can put additional strain on muscles.

Problem solve. I believe this step is often the most important and yet most frequently overlooked and one of the primary reasons I wrote this book. You will gain very little if you don't identify and eliminate the activities that repeatedly and often unknowingly cause irritation and injury.[17] This is where you get to be the detective. As a physical therapist, I am a detective for my patients. I often see people for a full hour and we identify contributing factors and find solutions for as many of the culprits as we can. Usually, we build a list of ten to twenty solutions. This section will give you ideas and tips so you can identify ways to overcome hurtful habits and allow your muscles to heal. Remember, all the causes of muscle pain and trigger points discussed at the beginning of this chapter can contribute to myofascial pain and should be considered, even if they are not mentioned specifically for each muscle. You also may find it helpful to keep a symptom diary to help you identify contributing factors, as discussed in Chapter 9.

Release, relax, stretch, and move. Stretching and healthy movement are usually essential steps in relieving the discomfort from tense, tender muscles. They can help you relax and also improve your function, which is important if, for example, you can't turn your head to back up your car safely. However, trigger point treatment is not the same for everyone and should be discussed with your healthcare provider and customized for you. For example, if you stretch a jaw that is locked, you can cause serious damage to the joint structures. Or, if you are hypermobile, stretching could make some joints more unstable. If you have jaw or neck-joint problems, it is important to understand the condition of your joints as well as any underlying conditions before starting a program. These problems could include—but are not limited to—arthritis, jaw clicking, locking, or cervical dysfunction. Others with fibromyalgia, under a lot of stress, or suffering from chronic pain conditions can be extremely sensitive to pressure and stretching and may need a customized program. My role is to introduce you to possibilities that you can discuss with your health-care provider and you can decide together what is best for you. In general, the goal is to find and release trigger points in order to relax, stretch, and safely move the muscle to restore length and function. Generally, stretching or lengthening of the muscle should be achieved before starting exercises that shorten or load the muscle. Stretching should feel good, as when you are finally able to straighten a leg you have been sitting on for a while. So if you have pain, you should stop. If a muscle is chronically tight or extremely tender, it may tolerate minimal stretching, whereas a relatively new trigger point in an otherwise healthy muscle will tolerate much more active stretching. I find it helpful to stretch my sorest side last. An ideal time to stretch is when your muscles are warm, like after exercise or in a warm shower. Think of your muscles like gum. If you want to stretch the gum enough to blow bubbles, you must first move (chew) and warm up the gum. There are many ways to release, relax, stretch, and move each muscle, but I have been conservative in the level of difficulty of the stretches I have picked and introduced only one or two for most muscles that you can discuss with your health-care provider and then do by yourself at home. If you do not have success, physical therapists and other professionals are specially trained in many fabulous techniques to assist you. However, fewer are trained in helping you identify the contributing factors. So pay close attention to the problem-solving sections.[18]

Trapezius Muscle

The material in this section is largely based on clinical experience and on the work of Fernández-de-Las-Peñas, Alonso-Blanco, Cuadrado, Gerwin, and Pareja;[19] Saunders;[20] and Simons, Travell, and Simons.[21]

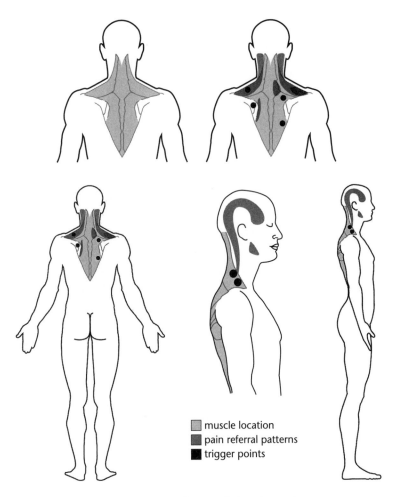

FIGURE 8.3: Trapezius muscle location, pain referral patterns, and trigger points

Location. The trapezius is a kite-shaped muscle, with the top of the kite at the back of your head, the pointy sides attaching to your shoulders, and the bottom of the kite attaching to your mid-back at the bottom of your thoracic spine (see Figure 8.3).

Pain referral and symptoms. Trigger points in this muscle can refer pain from the back of your skull, curving from behind your ear, to the side of your head (in the shape of a question mark). It can also refer pain from the middle of your back to the tips of your shoulders and into your neck. A trapezius trigger point can cause painful neck rotation and limit your ability to bend your ear to your opposite shoulder (see Figure 8.3).

Action. This muscle elevates the shoulders, pulls back and stabilizes the shoulder blades, and rotates the shoulder socket upward.

Problem solve. The following tips can help you resolve a trapezius muscle problem:

- Get a good chair with a supportive back and armrests. If you are in an occupation such as dentistry, drafting, or the like, or have short upper arms that don't reach typical armrests, try to arrange some type of arm support to periodically relieve the trapezius muscle. When sitting on a couch or chair, rest your arms on extra pillows or on a purse or backpack on your lap. When standing, unload the weight from this muscle by putting your hands in your pockets.

- Beware of lifting and carrying your purse or briefcase. Use a rolling bag or lighten your bag by buying multiple sets of the necessities you carry and leaving one set at the office or in the car. Hold your purse or bag against your body, close to your center of gravity behind your belly button. Reaching to place a purse or briefcase on the floor of the car's passenger seat every day puts a tremendous amount of stress on your neck and shoulder muscles. Place it in your trunk or behind you instead. Use a backpack with two straps or a waist strap to help distribute the weight.

- Avoid extra pressure directly on the muscle, such as that created by a tight bra or a purse or backpack strap. Sports bras and ones with narrow straps are common culprits. Try a bra with wide nonelastic straps or try moving the strap to the tip of the shoulder off the muscle.

- Arrange your computer workstation ergonomically. Adjust the keyboard and mouse so they are not so high that you have to elevate your shoulders to reach them. (For more information on setting up your workspace, see Figure 4.6 on page 54.)

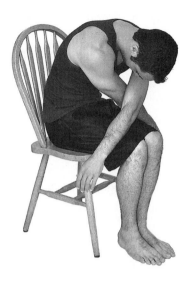

FIGURE 8.4: Crossover Arm Stretch

- Beware of whiplash-type injuries, including flicking your hair out of your eyes or rolling your head in circles.

- Use a headset or speakerphone when talking on your home, work, or cell phone. Do not clamp the phone to your ear by shrugging your shoulder up to your ear.

- Address postural asymmetries such as a leg-length discrepancy or hemipelvis.

Release, relax, stretch, and move. You often see people rubbing trigger points in their upper trapezius, but you will likely need a partner or trigger point instrument, such as a small ball in a pair of pantyhose held between your back and the wall to reach many of the trigger points in the mid and lower trapezius. You can apply the gentle pressure release techniques to the trigger points and massage or strum those areas. Note that the muscle fibers run in different directions. Before you stretch your trapezius muscle using the following exercises, you may want to stretch any tight pectoralis muscles discussed later in this chapter (see Figures 8.22 and 8.23 on page 164), which pull your shoulders into a rounded position and cause the trapezius muscle to tighten.

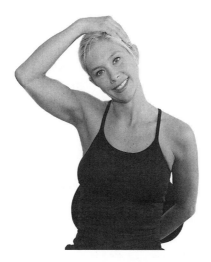

FIGURE 8.5: Ear-to-Shoulder Stretch

EXERCISE \ *Crossover Arm Stretch*

Sitting on a chair or stool so that your feet are firmly and comfortably on the floor, straighten your arms and cross them, so that your right arm is on the outside of your left thigh and vice versa. Then take a deep breath in, and as you exhale, slowly lower and hang your head allowing your body weight to gently cross your arms further (see Figure 8.4). Breathe in again and repeat two more times.

EXERCISE \ *Ear-to-Shoulder Stretch*

Start by sitting in a chair. Place your right hand on the left side of your head. Use your hand to gently tilt your right ear toward your right shoulder, letting your hand do all the work. Stop when you feel a gentle stretch in the muscles on the left side of your neck. Stay in your comfort range and hold for five to ten seconds, and repeat three to four times, as needed. Reverse sides and repeat with your right hand moving your left ear toward your left shoulder (see Figure 8.5). It may be helpful to stretch your tighter side last. To make the stretch easier, you can do this exercise lying on your back. As you progress, you can increase the stretch by placing your free left hand behind your back or anchoring it at the base of the chair to create a pull in the opposite direction of the stretch.

You can also try this stretch in the upright position. I love to do it in a warm shower. Then maintain your mobility with movement like the relaxation shoulder rolls described below, or using other appropriate activities. Swimming can be ideal for maintaining the mobility of the trapezius, but start slowly. Jarring activities like jogging may aggravate the trapezius muscle.

EXERCISE \ *Relaxation Shoulder Rolls*

This is a way to gently move and relax the trapezius and related neck and shoulder muscles. Sit or stand with your arms hanging loosely by your sides and pretend that you are going to draw circles with the tips of your shoulders. The circles should be relaxed. The movement should feel good. Spend 10 to 15 seconds rotating your shoulders clockwise, and then repeat, rotating them counterclockwise. You may notice some noise or gentle popping. This is a common occurrence but should not be painful or problematic. Usually slowing down helps. As always, discuss any concerns with your health-care provider.

Sternocleidomastoid Muscle (SCM)

The material in this section is largely based on clinical experience and the work of Fernández-de-Las-Peñas, Alonso-Blanco, Cuadrado, Gerwin, and Pareja;[22] Saunders;[23] Travell and Simons;[24] and Simons, Travell, and Simons.[25]

Location. The SCM attaches just behind your ear and splits into two parts. The sternal part attaches to the top of your sternum and the clavicular part to your clavicle (see Figure 8.6).

Pain referral and symptoms. Trigger points in the SCM can cause tension headaches that can easily be mistaken for a vascular-type migraine headache, and these types of tension headaches have an incredibly complex pain and symptom pattern. SCM dysfunction can cause postural dizziness that can be almost debilitating. You can experience problems turning your head or glancing downward. It can cause neck pain, pain in the upper sternum, and a feeling that the glands in your neck are swollen, as well as pain on the top of your head. You can have earaches and frontal headaches, and pain can be referred to the face and sinuses. People with SCM trigger points can

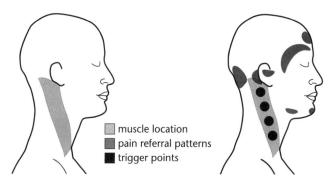

FIGURE 8.6: Sternocleidomastoid muscle location, pain referral patterns, and trigger points

even complain of blurred vision, excessive production of tears, sore throat, dry cough, and ringing in the ears.[26]

Action. Together, the two sides of the SCM flex the neck forward and can help in breathing. Each side works by itself to help rotate your face to the opposite side. The SCM muscle helps lift your head when you are getting up from lying on your back or side.

Problem solve. The following tips can help you avoid common contributing factors to myofascial pain and dysfunction of the SCM:

- Watching TV or a screen turned at an awkward angle is a common cause. Place your computer monitor or TV screen straight in front of you. At the computer, use a document holder so you don't have to turn your head for prolonged periods. Beware of activities that require repeated neck rotation or head rolling, like swimming.

- Avoid clamping the phone to your ear with your shoulder. Use a headset or speakerphone.

- Avoid reading in bed with a light on one side. This setup tends to cause you to turn your head for prolonged periods. Put the light overhead or listen to books on tape.

- Beware of whiplash-type injuries, even those possibly caused by something as simple as a roller coaster–type ride or flipping your hair.

- Breathe through your nose and use your diaphragm. Breathing with your mouth open and chest rising, instead of through your nose and using your diaphragm, can cause the SCM to overwork.

- Sleep with a cervical pillow that does not push your head forward, but fits the curves of your neck. Pull the sides of the pillow around you to prevent your head from being turned or rotated all night, which can irritate the SCM.

- Beware of overhead activities such as painting, hanging curtains, or sitting in the front row at the theatre.

- Assess for asymmetries like a leg-length discrepancy or short upper arms.

- Hangover headaches, chronic infections (e.g., tooth abscesses), and spinal tap headaches can irritate this muscle group. Resolve these health concerns with the appropriate professional.

- Adjust the headrest in cars and elsewhere where it may be pushing your head forward.

- Loosen your neckties and shirt collars so they don't press on the SCM.

- When rolling over in bed, roll your head on your pillow instead of lifting your head. When getting out of bed, try lifting your head with the non-sore side up instead of lifting it straight off the pillow, which can aggravate the SCM.

Release, relax, stretch, and move. To help locate your SCM, try turning your head to the right. The sternal part of the left SCM should feel like a strap that starts under your ear and runs down to your sternum. You can find and release trigger points and then stretch and gently move the SCM, using the following exercises:

EXERCISE   *The Rolling Nod*

This is one of my favorite neck exercises to gently move your neck, and it can be performed in several positions: sitting, standing, or lying on your back. If you are lying down, you can reduce friction by placing a thin, slippery book under your head. Gently nod your head, using small upward and downward movements. While you are nodding, rotate your head slowly from left to right. When you reach the end of your range of motion or you feel a gentle pull, hold and nod five times, then slowly nod and rotate in the opposite direction. Don't forget to breathe, and if you are out in public, smile at any people next to you who might be wondering why in the world you are nodding your head.

We have opted not to include stretches that more specifically isolate this muscle group since it can be especially sensitive and some stretching motions can potentially occlude or pinch an artery in your neck, which can be problematic for a small group of people. You will stretch various parts of this complex muscle if you perform some of the other stretches mentioned in this chapter, like the "Ear-to-Shoulder Stretch" (see Figure 8.5 on page 139), "Hands-Behind-Head Stretch" (see Figure 8.14 on page 154), and "Rotatation, Chin-to-Shoulder Stretch" (see Figure 8.18 on page 159). As always, check with your health-care providers before starting a new exercise routine and discontinue it if you have any adverse or unusual symptoms.

Temporalis Muscle

The material in this section is largely based on clinical experience and the work of Fernández-de-Las-Peñas, Alonso-Blanco, Cuadrado, Gerwin, and Pareja;[27] Travell and Simons;[28] and Simons, Travell, and Simons.[29]

Location. The temporalis is a fan-shaped muscle that covers your scalp in the area of your temples, from behind the eye to just above and behind your ear, and it has fibers running upward and downward to a common attachment on the coronoid process of the mandible (see Figure 8.7 on the next page).

Pain referral and symptoms. Trigger points in this muscle are a common cause of headaches and pain in the front and sides of the head and occasionally the jaw joint. Temporalis muscle dysfunction can cause pain behind the eye and in the eyebrow region, as well as hypersensitivity of the upper jaw and upper teeth. When you open and close your mouth, muscular tightness and imbalances can make this uncoordinated and asymmetrical. Your teeth may feel like they don't fit together right or you may be sensitive to hot and cold or have

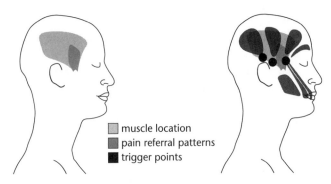

FIGURE 8.7: Temporalis muscle location, pain
referral patterns, and trigger points

diffuse pain when you bite down. You may not want to have your
teeth filed down or pulled or have a root canal done unless you are
sure that a trigger point is not the true cause of your tooth pain.

Action. The primary action of the temporalis muscle is to close the
mouth. Both sides can help pull the chin backward and one side can
pull the lower jaw to the same side.

Problem solve. The following tips can help you resolve a temporalis
problem:

- Address a forward head posture, postural asymmetries, and
  sleeping posture.

- Tone and train your tongue to rest on the roof of your mouth,
  which helps the jaw muscles relax.

- Avoid exhaustive clenching or grinding of teeth, chewing, and
  biting.

- Beware of prolonged overopening, like would be required during a lengthy dental procedure.

- Avoid chill stress caused by a cold draft. Try wearing a scarf or
  hood or even sleeping with a loose nightcap if your temporalis
  muscle is stressed by cold.

- Eliminate mouth breathing, clenching, and grinding at night
  and other problems with your bite. You may benefit from an
  occlusal splint.

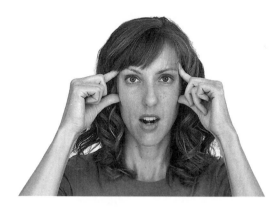

FIGURE 8.8: Orbiting with Finger Lengthening of Temples

- Look for and eliminate any trapezius and sternocleidomastoid trigger points, which are often associated with the temporalis muscle.

- As always, address any other causes of muscle pain and trigger points discussed at the beginning of this chapter.

Release, relax, stretch and move. You can palpate for and release trigger points in the temporalis best when your jaw is relaxed and slightly open. You can stretch the temporalis muscle by using the following exercise.

EXERCISE   *Orbiting with Finger Lengthening of Temples*

Orbiting is my favorite jaw stretch and exercise (also in Chapter 6) to gently stretch the muscles that brace, clench, and grind, including the temporalis. Start with the front third of your tongue on the roof of your mouth, in a resting position. Keeping the front third of your tongue on the roof of your mouth, gently open and close your mouth in the pain-free and click-free range. To help improve the lengthening of the temporalis, you can place the soft pads of your fingers on your temples and apply gentle pressure upward along the fibers of the muscle as you breathe in. If you get the okay from your health-care provider, you can increase the stretch by keeping only the tip of your tongue—instead of the front third—on the roof of your mouth. Repeat three to five times as needed. Remember, never force a locked joint to open and always check with your specialist if you have joint abnormalities or any concerns (see Figure 8.8).

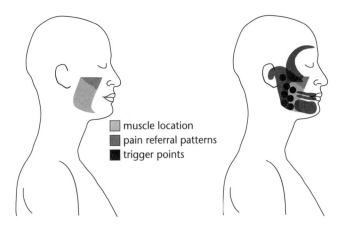

FIGURE 8.9: Masseter muscle location, pain referral patterns, and trigger points

Masseter Muscle

The material in this section is largely based on clinical experience and on the work of Ono et al.;[30] Travell and Simons;[31] and Simons, Travell, and Simons.[32]

Location. The masseter extends from the angle of your lower jaw, or mandible, up to your maxilla and cheekbone, or zygomatic arch (see Figure 8.9).

Pain referral and symptoms. The majority of people with TMJ disorders have trigger points in this muscle, which can cause pain in the area of the upper and lower jaw and molar teeth; the TMJ; the ears (e.g., ringing in one ear); the eyebrows; and under the eyes (e.g., restricted blood flow below the eyes, causing stuffiness or bags under the eyes).

Action. The primary action of the masseter muscle is to close the mouth. The masseter and temporalis both close the mouth. The masseter does more of the chewing while the temporalis does more of the postural positioning and balancing. The masseter also has some deep fibers that help to retrude, or pull in, the chin.

Problem solve. The following tips can help resolve a masseter trigger point problem:

- Correct a forward head posture during your day and night activities.

- Eliminate mouth breathing, close your lips, anchor your tongue on "the spot," and establish a healthy posture of the jaw with your teeth apart.

- Stop clenching and grinding your teeth. Avoid sustained pressure caused by holding things between your teeth (e.g., a pencil) or biting your fingernails.

- Eliminate chewy, painful, or tiring foods and items such as gum, nuts, and ice, and learn to swallow correctly.

- Thoroughly evaluate teeth that contact prematurely. Make sure there is a true bite problem. If your bite was thrown off immediately after getting a new crown or filling, this is likely the culprit. However, a bite that seems to change "out of the blue" is likely caused by a muscular imbalance or joint dysfunction and should be treated accordingly.

- Treat related trigger points (e.g., the SCM and trapezius).

- Beware of traumatic or long dental procedures. Take breaks during the procedure or schedule multiple appointments.

- Treat joint problems and tooth or gum infections.

- Reduce stressors that can increase muscle tension. This would be helpful for most muscles. However, some, like the masseter, harbor tension more easily.

- Avoid the physical stress of lifting heavy objects, because people usually clench their teeth when they strain.

- Avoid immobilization, which can shorten and irritate this muscle.

- Watch for deficiencies in thyroid, vitamins, minerals, and electrolytes.

- An occlusal splint made and worn correctly can be very beneficial in restoring normal muscle balance and occlusion.

Release, relax, stretch, and move. You can more easily find your masseter if you clench your teeth. You can feel it tighten under your

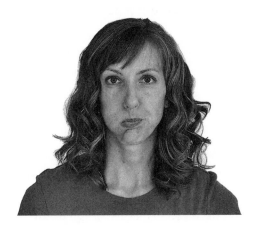

FIGURE 8.10: The Lopsided Blowfish

fingers over the angle of your lower jaw, making it easy to palpate for and to release trigger points. You can stretch your masseter muscle using the orbiting exercise (as seen in Figure 5.1 on page 78 and Figure 8.8 on page 145). You can also try The Lopsided Blowfish (see Figure 8.10, described below). This exercise is especially effective after melting masseter trigger points with gentle pressure release or strumming the muscle.

EXERCISE \ *The Lopsided Blowfish*

You can stretch the masseter using the orbiting stretch discussed above. You can also relax and stretch the masseter by blowing air into your cheeks. You can fill both cheeks with air at the same time or stretch just one cheek at a time, like a lopsided blowfish (see Figure 8.10). Hold for three to five seconds and repeat as needed.

The Lateral Pterygoid

The material in this section is largely based on clinical experience and the work of Simons, Travell, and Simons (1999).[33]

Location. This muscle is located on the inside upper portion of the TMJ (see Figure 8.11). There are two parts to this muscle: an upper superior head and a lower inferior head. The superior head of this muscle attaches to the front of the joint capsule where the disk attaches.

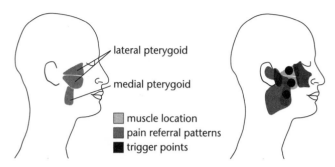

FIGURE 8.11: Lateral and medial pterygoid muscle location, pain referral patterns, and trigger points

Pain referral and symptoms. Trigger points in this muscle project pain to the TMJ and maxilla and can adversely alter your bite and temporomandibular joint function. This perceived "joint pain" is often misinterpreted as pain from arthritis.

Action. The superior head of the lateral pterygoid often attaches to the TMJ capsule and articular disk.[34] The inferior head pulls your chin or mandible forward, downward, and toward the opposite side.

Problem solve. The following tips can help you correct the common causes of a lateral pterygoid problem:

- An occlusal splint may be needed to help prevent or eliminate touching teeth and provide stability to let the muscles calm down, so you can restore your normal bite. The splint must be properly fitted, and modifications may need to be made along the way.

- Improve your posture, as discussed in Chapter 4. Directly or indirectly, posture affects all of the muscles we will discuss. This includes addressing asymmetries such as a leg-length difference. Also, you need to ensure correct sleeping posture. If you are a side sleeper, be sure your head and jaw are lightly supported.

- Anchor your tongue on the roof of your mouth and work to close your lips and separate your teeth.

- Avoid trauma or strains to the jaw, which can particularly affect this muscle.

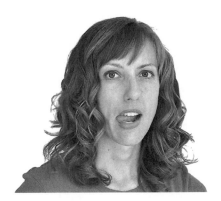

FIGURE 8.12: Tongue Waggle

- Don't chew gum or ice and/or grind your teeth.
- Decrease the hyperirritability of the central nervous system by eliminating clenching or stress and breathing deeply through your nose and with your diaphragm.
- If you have "joint pain," yet are told your joint looks fine, this muscle is often the cause.
- Watch for low levels of B vitamins and folic acid, which can increase irritability.

Release, relax, stretch and move. You can feel for and release trigger points in the lateral pterygoid using a cleaned hand or a gloved finger and reaching inside your mouth to the upper back corner inside of your cheek. If you don't want to put your hands into your mouth, you may feel a tiny piece of it by sliding your finger along the lower part of the cheekbone. As you slide from your ear toward your nose, your finger will drop into a gully. Right where your finger dropped you may feel a piece of the lateral pterygoid. Because the lateral pterygoid muscle is so intricately tied to the TMJ, any stretching should be done cautiously and be guided by a TMJ expert. You can decrease the tension in your lateral pterygoid muscles by orbiting with a mirror (see Figure 5.1 on page 78). A tight pterygoid muscle can pull the lower jaw to one side on opening, so go slowly and focus on trying to open using a vertically straight movement. You can also help the muscle relax by using the following exercise.

> EXERCISE \ ***Tongue Waggle***
>
> Let your jaw completely relax and hang slightly open while you waggle your tongue from side to side. This can be done while sitting or lying down (see Figure 8.12).

The Medial Pterygoid

The material in this section is largely based on clinical experience and on the work of Travell and Simons[35] *and Simons, Travell, and Simons.*[36]

Location. This muscle is located below and inside the lower angle of the mandible (see Figure 8.11 on page 149).

Pain referral and symptoms. Trigger points in this muscle can project pain to the back of the mouth and throat. Pain can also be referred behind and below the TMJ, and deep inside the ear. Trigger points in this muscle can limit and cause deviation in opening and indirectly cause ear stuffiness and painful swallowing.

Action. The primary actions are to move the chin or mandible toward the opposite side, upward, and forward.

Problem solve. The following tips can help you resolve a medial pterygoid problem:

- Correct postural problems, including gently supporting the jaw during side sleeping so it isn't pulling to the side all night.
- Eliminate hurtful jaw habits, including teeth grinding.
- Use of an occlusal splint may be necessary.
- Decrease physical and emotional stressors.
- Treat chronic infections, such as herpes simplex.
- Treat associated trigger points. Check the lateral pterygoid and masseter.

Release, relax, stretch, and move. You can best find and release the trigger points by using a gloved finger or clean hand, and feeling for tenderness inside your mouth behind your last molar tooth. Since this muscle is inside the TMJ, you may only feel a small part of it on the outside of your mouth if you slightly open your mouth and palpate the inside corner of the angle of your lower jaw. You can inhibit tension in your medial pterygoid muscle by using the "Tongue Waggle" exercise (see Figure 8.12 on page 150) and the "Orbiting with and Without a Mirror" exercise (see Figure 5.1 on page 78). Because the pterygoid muscles are interrelated and connected with the joint, any direct stretching should be performed cautiously and only by a TMJ expert who has evaluated your joint.

Digastric Muscle

The material in this section is largely based on clinical experience, a study by Ono et al. (2009),[37] and the work of Travell and Simons[38] and Simons, Travell, and Simons.[39]

Location. The digastric muscle has two parts. The back part attaches behind the ear and the front part attaches under the chin. The two parts join together on the hyoid bone, which is located just above your larynx, to form a sling (see Figure 8.13).

Pain referral and symptoms. Trigger points in this muscle can cause painful swallowing. The muscle refers pain to the bottom four middle incisor teeth and the upper part of the SCM. In fact, you may think the pain is caused by the SCM, even if it is really caused by the digastric muscle.

Action. The primary action is to open the mouth and stabilize the hyoid bone. The digastric muscle also plays an important role in swallowing.

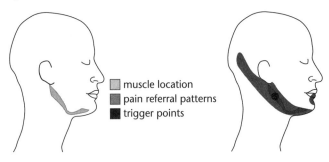

■ muscle location
■ pain referral patterns
■ trigger points

FIGURE 8.13: Digastric muscle location, pain referral patterns, and trigger points

Problem solve. The following tips can help you resolve a digastric muscle problem:

- Learn to swallow correctly.
- Address postural problems as previously discussed.
- Breathe through your nose. Eliminate mouth breathing.
- Avoid the sources of whiplash-type injuries, including things like stressful roller coaster rides.
- Stop grinding your teeth.
- Address trigger points in the masseter and other muscles that close the mouth.

Release, relax, stretch, and move. Because the digastric muscle has two bellies, or parts, you need to palpate two areas for trigger point identification and management. Lying on your back with your mouth closed and your head extended as if you are looking upward slightly, palpate the first spot just under the front of your chin on either side of the midline. You are actually stretching part of the digastric muscle in this position as well, and you can gently strum it along its muscle fibers. You can also stretch the front of the neck and portions of the digastric muscle with the "Hands-Behind-Head Stretch" described below.

> EXERCISE \ *Hands-Behind-Head Stretch*
>
> While sitting in a chair with a back support and with your hands interlaced behind and supporting your neck, gently bend your head backward until you feel a gentle stretch under the chin and at the front of your neck (see Figure 8.14 on the next page). Go very slowly and gently. If you feel dizzy or have any discomfort or unusual symptoms, discontinue the stretch. As always, check with your doctor if you have any concerns. This movement can also gently stretch portions of the sternocleidomastoid and other muscles in the neck. The second spot is more difficult to palpate, or stretch, and it is found just behind the angle of your jaw, below your ear but in front of your sternocleidomastoid muscle.

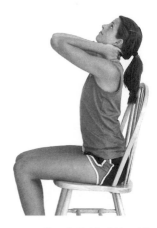

FIGURE 8.14: Hands-Behind-Head Stretch

Middle and Deep Muscles at the Back of Your Neck: Semispinalis Capitis and Cervicis, Multifidi and Rotatores
The material in this section is largely based on clinical experience and on the work of Travell and Simons[40] and Simons, Travell, and Simons.[41]

Location. The posterior cervical muscles make up most of the middle and deep layers beneath your trapezius muscle and along your upper spine. They run up to the back of your skull and along your upper neck and shoulder girdle in various directions. Because of the number and location of these muscles, we will illustrate only the primary trigger points and pain referral patterns for them (see Figure 8.15).

Pain referral and symptoms. Trigger points in these muscles can cause pain that feels like a tight headband just above your eyes and tenderness on the back of your head. They can cause headaches; irritate the back of the head, neck, and shoulders; and entrap the occipital nerve, leading to an occipital neuralgia, which is an irritation of the occipital nerves at the base of the skull.[42] An irritated nerve in your cervical spine often irritates these muscles as well. Someone with a long neck is prone to the irritation of these muscles. Tightness in these muscles can limit forward bending and rotation of the head and neck.

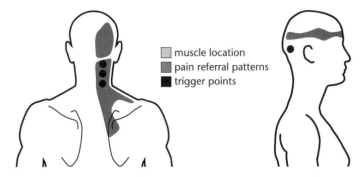

FIGURE 8.15: Posterior cervical muscle location,
pain referral patterns, and trigger points

Action. These muscles primarily rotate, stabilize, and facilitate the backward bend of your head and neck.

Problem solve. The following tips can help you eliminate causes or perpetuators of a posterior cervical muscle problem:

- Avoid reading or watching TV on your stomach or propped up on your elbows.

- An ice pack at the base of the skull can help calm irritated occipital nerves (see Chapters 10 and 12).

- Avoid a forward head posture. Do not bend your head forward when performing activities such as typing, computing, reading, writing, sewing, or playing music. Try stacking pillows on your lap or use a reading or music stand to bring what you are doing up closer toward you. Stretching the posterior cervical muscles is an important part of restoring a balanced head posture.

- Beware of falls, whiplash injuries, and trauma to this area.

- Avoid tight collars or caps that can irritate or constrict these muscles.

- Adjust your eyewear. If your eyeglass lenses are tilted incorrectly, adjust them so you do not feel the need to bend forward.

- These muscles are often irritated by joint problems, including arthritis, nerve, and inflammatory disorders.

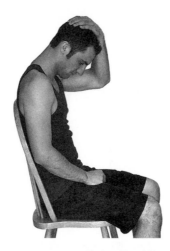

FIGURE 8.16: Sitting Head Hang

- Treat symptoms of depression. Depression can particularly irritate this muscle group,[43] perhaps because depressed individuals tend to slouch and round their shoulders. The pectoralis muscle is also often tight due to constant slouching and this should be addressed.

- Arrange your computer workstation ergonomically (see Figure 4.6 on page 54).

- Sleep with your head supported appropriately and avoid tilting your head backward. Keep it level, neutral, and balanced.

Release, relax, stretch, and move. Stretch your posterior cervical muscles using the following exercise. In addition, stretching your pectoralis major muscles (see Figures 8.22 and 8.23 on pages 164 and 165) can be helpful. Remember, all stretches and exercises should be approved by your health-care provider, particularly if you have a known health concern or condition.

EXERCISE \ *Sitting Head Hang*

Sit on a comfortable chair and lean forward. With your head bent forward and your hand or hands positioned lightly on top of your head, as you breathe in, look down and gently pull your chin toward your chest as you breathe out. Let your head sink and let your back gently stretch (see Figure 8.16). This feels especially wonderful if you can do it in a warm shower or sitting on a chair. To stretch the rotational fibers of the muscle, you need to look downward while you slightly rotate your chin toward one shoulder at a time while also applying gentle pressure with your hand on the top of your head. Be extremely gentle. Remember that if you are sensitive to stretching or have cervical dysfunction, you should check with your health-provider for alternatives. You can often gain some neck motion simply by moving your eyes in the direction toward which you want to stretch, so there are varying levels and methods of stretching.

Splenius Capitis and Splenius Cervicis

The material in this section is largely based on clinical experience and on the work of Travell and Simons[44] and Simons, Travell, and Simons.[45]

Location. The splenius muscles lie under the trapezius and semispinalis muscles. The splenius capitis runs from the lower cervical and upper thoracic vertebrae up to the base of the skull. The splenius cervicis attaches to the vertebrae just below the capitis, wrapping upward and around the splenius capitis to attach to the outer lateral parts of the vertebrae (see Figure 8.17).

Pain referral and symptoms. Trigger points in these muscles can cause pain on the top of your head, just behind your eyes, and at the

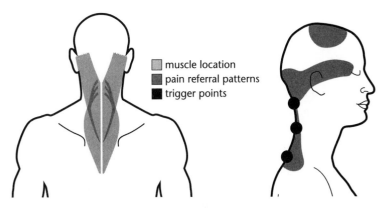

muscle location
pain referral patterns
trigger points

FIGURE 8.17: Splenius capitis and cervicis muscle location, pain referral patterns, and trigger points

angle of your neck, where your shoulders and neck come together. They can also cause headaches, neck pain, and blur your vision.

Action. These muscles primarily rotate your neck and allow it to bend backward.

Problem solve. The following tips can help you eliminate causes or perpetuators of splenius muscle problems:

- Avoid positions where your head is rotated and tilted slightly upward. This can occur when sleeping without appropriate pillow support, with your head bent backward or rotated in an awkward situation, on the couch with your head on the armrest, or while sitting on the floor with your arms on your knees and looking slightly upward.

- When pulling weights or ropes, be careful not to rotate or project your head forward.

- Whiplash injuries cause and contribute to problems in these muscles.

- Arrange your computer workstation ergonomically, paying close attention to avoid having your head turned, as may occur when you attempt to view a poorly placed screen or document.

- Musicians should avoid awkward or irritating head positions.

- Cold temperatures can particularly irritate these muscles and care must be taken to keep them warm.

- Cervical and thoracic joint dysfunction can contribute to splenius trigger points.

Release, relax, stretch, and move. The stretch for these muscles is similar to the Sitting Head-Hang Stretch described above for use in exercising the posterior cervical muscles.

EXERCISE \ *Rotation, Chin-to-Shoulder Head-Hang Stretch*

In this exercise you will place your hand on the back of your head and gently rotate your face and pull your chin toward the same-side shoulder. Stretch both directions through your painfree range (see Figure 8.18).

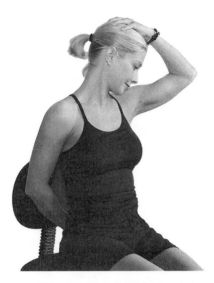

FIGURE 8.18: Rotation, Chin-to-Shoulder Head-Hang Stretch

Suboccipitals—Muscles Below the Back of the Skull

The material in this section is largely based on clinical experience and on the work of Fernández-de-las-Peñas, Alonso-Blanco, Cuadrado, Gerwin, and Pareja[46] *and Simons, Travell, and Simons.*[47]

Location. The suboccipital muscles include several small muscles that run in various directions at the base of your skull (see Figure 8.19 on the next page) and are a common cause of headaches. They are located deep beneath several other muscles, so they are difficult to palpate and can radiate pain from the base of the skull upward behind the ear to the eye.

Pain referral and symptoms. These muscles can cause enough discomfort at the base of the skull that it becomes painful to rest the back of your head on a pillow. Problems with these muscles can cause headaches and restrict your ability to look downward, move your ear toward your same-side shoulder, or turn your head in order to see well enough to back out your car or check your blind spot.

Action. These muscles also move your skull. They allow you to bend your skull backward and to rotate and tilt your head to each side.

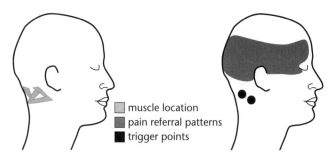

FIGURE 8.19: Suboccipital muscle location, pain
referral patterns, and trigger points

Problem solve. The following can help you correct a suboccipital muscle problem:

- Fix your posture: If you are a slouch-a-holic but you don't want to continually stare at the floor, you chronically contract these tiny muscles to level your eyes and head. After trying the "Posture Quick Fix" (see page 46), you may need to add the "Chin Tuck" exercise described on the next page to help you level your head. Adjust your sleeping posture as needed, because people with suboccipital pain can find it uncomfortable to lie on their back without some accommodations.

- Beware of anything that requires you to look upward, rotate, or awkwardly position your head for long periods. Don't sit in the front row during movies or plays. Don't perform work over your head, like painting a ceiling. Even repeatedly tilting your head to drink from a cup or can may irritate these muscles.

- Avoid trifocal glasses or inverted bifocals because they require minute movements of the head that can irritate the suboccipitals.

- Make sure your television or computer screen is not positioned too high.

- Cold temperatures can irritate these muscles, especially at night. Wear a scarf, redirect the air conditioning vents, or wear your hair down.

Release, relax, stretch, and move. Because of their location and attachments, only a trained professional using special manual techniques can differentiate between the suboccipital muscles and the posterior cervical muscles and specifically treat them. Often the cervical spine is involved and requires treatment as well. Once treated, the professional may choose to have you elongate your suboccipital muscles, using the following exercise. You can also gently move these muscles with The Rolling Nod in a sitting position, making sure to tuck your head as you go.

EXERCISE \ *Chin Tuck*

While sitting or standing in a comfortable and balanced neutral posture, tuck your chin backward and upward as if you were making a double chin, while simultaneously lifting and elongating the back of your head. Many people perform this exercise by pushing the chin with their hand, but as this loads the jaw joint, I prefer to use my imagination or to do it actively by gently pressing upward and backward below the nose (see Figure 8.20).

EXERCISE \ *Suboccipital Release*

A physical therapist can perform a manual suboccipital release that feels magical. Since I am trained in how to perform this manual suboccipital release, my teenage daughter begs me to do this to her at night after she has had a long day. This release can melt the tension at the base of the skull, and when combined with a gentle stretch, it feels much like your head is floating on a wave moving farther out to sea. It is gentle but effective.

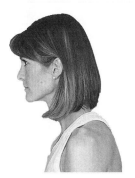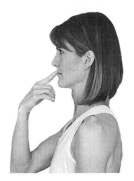

FIGURE 8.20: Chin Tuck

Pectoralis Major ("Slouch-a-Holic Muscle")

The material in this section is largely based on clinical experience and on the work of Travell and Simons[48] *and Simons, Travell, and Simons.*[49]

Location. The pectoralis muscles are your main chest muscles. The pectoralis major is the largest and closest muscle to the surface, attaching along your sternum at the middle of your chest and gathering into bands that attach to your upper arm (see Figure 8.21).

Pain referral and symptoms. This muscle group can cause pain in the chest, shoulder, arm, and fingers. Your breast may be sore or your nipple hypersensitive, making it difficult to wear a bra or shirt. These muscles can indirectly cause pain in the mid-back because rounded shoulders due to tight pectoralis muscles strain the back. The muscles can even cause symptoms that mimic heart disease. The opposite is true as well: These muscles can be irritated by heart disease. It is critical to have any chest pain properly evaluated.

Action. The primary movements allow you to bring your arm close to your side, pull your arm across your chest, and rotate your arm inward. When these muscles are tight, they pull the shoulders forward,

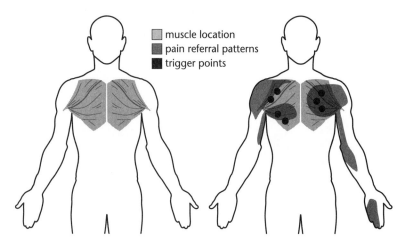

muscle location
pain referral patterns
trigger points

FIGURE 8.21: Pectoralis major muscle location, pain referral patterns, and trigger points

resulting in rounded shoulders with a stooped-forward head posture.

Problem solve. The following tips can help you correct pectoralis muscle problems:

- Improve your posture. Mentally, sign up for slouch-a-holics anonymous by reviewing the steps outlined in Chapter 4.

- Avoid sleeping on your side, which shortens the pectoralis muscle group you are lying on, especially since most people let their up arm fall across their chest, shortening that pectoralis group as well. Do not sleep on your back with your arms crossed against the body or touching your face. I can often tell which side people sleep on or cross against their body by which shoulder is more slouched or rounded. If you have to sleep on your side, try placing a pillow under your ribs on the downward side, creating a pocket for your shoulder, as described in Chapter 4, and placing a pillow under the arm on the top side to keep gravity from crossing the arm against your body.

- Relax and lengthen the pectoralis muscles by opening your chest, employing good posture and proper stretching. Sometimes swelling in the arms can be caused by the fibers of this muscle group entrapping the lymph nodes, and this can be improved if the muscle is relaxed and lengthened.

- Avoid heavy lifting and sustained holding or reaching motions, such as clipping the hedges, using a chain saw, or sailing a boat.

Release, relax, stretch, and move. You can easily palpate the pectoralis major muscle by lifting your arms sideways so it is level with your shoulder. This position is most comfortable while lying on your back. With your thumb on the front of your armpit and the other fingers positioned opposite on the inside front part of your armpit, you can gently press your fingers together, feeling for trigger points and tightness. There are several ways you can stretch, relax, and move the pectoralis, including the following exercises and the Relaxation Shoulder Rolls described on page 140.

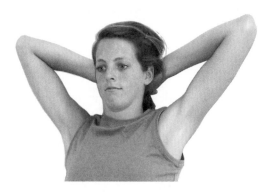

FIGURE 8.22: The Butterfly Stretch

EXERCISE \ *The Butterfly Stretch*

Lying comfortably on your back, interlock your fingers behind your head and neck so your elbows fan out like butterfly wings. Then bring your elbows backward toward the bed until you feel a gentle stretch in the chest (see Figure 8.22). As always, check with your health-care provider if you have shoulder problems or any other concerning condition.

EXERCISE \ *Hands-Behind-Back Stretch*

This is one of my favorite stretches to use after working on the computer or carrying things. It combines a stretch of the arm with a pectoralis stretch. While standing, hold your hands together behind your back, keeping your elbows straight. Some patients are so tight that they can not straighten their arms. This is okay, and you should only go to the point where you feel a gentle stretch in your pectoral muscles in the front of your chest (see Figure 8.23) and in the front of your arms. You can increase the stretch by spreading your chest to make your shoulder blades touch (as if you were holding an orange between your shoulder blades; see Figure 8.23).

Fibromyalgia

Fibromyalgia can be extremely frustrating and is common in people with TMJ disorders. People suffering from fibromyalgia and other muscle disorders may look healthy and normal, which can lead their

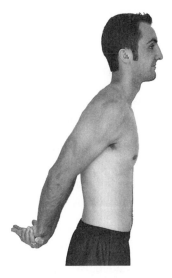

FIGURE 8.23: Hands-Behind-Back Stretch

family, friends, and even health-care providers to think it is "all in their head."

Fibromyalgia literally means pain of the muscles and other fibrous tissues. According to the American College of Rheumatology, "Fibromyalgia is a clinical syndrome defined by chronic widespread muscular pain, fatigue, and tenderness. Many people with fibromyalgia also experience additional symptoms such as fatigue, headaches, irritable bowel syndrome, irritable bladder, cognitive and memory problems (often called 'fibro fog'), temporomandibular joint disorder, pelvic pain, restless leg syndrome, sensitivity to noise and temperature, and anxiety and depression. These symptoms can vary in intensity and, like the pain of fibromyalgia, wax and wane over time."[50] Many, including fibromyalgia expert Dr. Devin Starlanyl (with Copeland), believe the nervous system in people with this condition works in overdrive, causing oversensitivity to smells, sounds, lights, pain, pressure, temperature fluctuations, and vibrations.[51]

According to the American College of Rheumatology, fibromyalgia affects 2 to 4 percent of the population.[52] It is estimated that 75 percent of people with fibromyalgia also have problems with their temporomandibular joints. Because 18 percent of people with TMJ disorders develop fibromyalgia, it is an important syndrome to understand. It affects more women than men.[53]

To receive a fibromyalgia diagnosis, after other possible causes are ruled out, you must usually meet two criteria:[54]

1. You must have widespread pain in all four quadrants of your body, lasting for at least three months.

2. You must have pain (not just tenderness) in at least eleven of the eighteen specified areas in Figure 8.24, when pressed with the pad of your thumb or forefinger at about 4 kg of pressure, which is enough to cause your nail bed to blanch, or turn white.

It is not uncommon for fibromyalgia patients to suffer for five years before receiving a diagnosis. Fibromyalgia is classified as a form of arthritis, so a rheumatologist who specializes in fibromyalgia can rule out any chemical or hormonal imbalances or other important concerns.

According to Dr. Robert Gerwin, a leading neurologist and pain expert, fibromyalgia and myofascial pain syndrome are a common

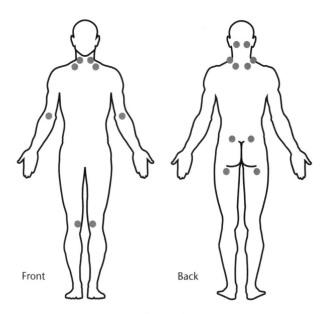

Front   Back

FIGURE 8.24: Fibromyalgia pain points

problem all over the world. The problem is not in diagnosing the condition, but in identifying the underlying causes and in developing an appropriate treatment plan. According to Dr. Gerwin, structural causes include scoliosis, joints that are insufficiently mobile, and overly loose joints. Metabolic causes include depleted iron, hypothyroidism, and vitamin D deficiency. Sometimes correcting one of these underlying causes is all that is needed to relieve the pain.[55]

People with fibromyalgia and myofascial pain can benefit from the healthy habits taught in this book; however, all should consult with a doctor before starting any exercise, stretching, or trigger point treatment program since their muscles and tissues can be extremely sensitive to pressure and stretching and every individual is different.

Summary

Now that you understand that muscles and connective tissue problems, called myofascial pain and dysfunction, can cause and perpetuate head, neck, and jaw pain and TMJ-related disorders, let's review some of the main points:

1. Myofascial pain is probably one of the most common and overlooked causes of head, neck, and jaw pain and dysfunction.

2. Even medical practitioners who are trained to treat myofascial pain often neglect to help the patient identify and eliminate causes and contributing factors, often leading to short-term relief and the need for repeated treatments.

3. This chapter can help to open your eyes and mind to possible causes of some of your symptoms and empower you with the tools to eliminate or alter those hurtful habits that are adding to your pain and dysfunction.

4. Talk with your health-care specialist about what type of exercise and stretching program is best for you.

5. People who suffer from fibromyalgia often have TMJ-related disorders.

6. Make yourself a checklist for change. Use Table 8.2 on the following page, which contains hypothetical examples, as a guide.

Table 8.2: Checklist for Change: Care for Your Muscles

HURTFUL HABIT	HEALTHY HABIT	CHECKLIST FOR CHANGE
I have ear pain, but my ear, nose, and throat doctor and TMJ expert say my ear and jaw joint are fine. Maybe the ear pain is caused by chewing gum, biting my nails, or grinding my teeth at night.	Decrease ear and joint pain; eliminate hurtful habits like gum chewing and nail biting.	I will buy dissolvable breath strips instead of chewing gum. I will cut my nails and paint them with clear, sour polish. I will problem solve the potential hurtful habits for the lateral pterygoid, masseter, sternocleidomastoid, and medial pterygoid. I will talk to my TMJ dentist about an occlusal splint.
I have pain in the back of my head and temporal headaches that may be from trigger points in my trapezius muscle, and sternocleido-mastoid muscles. It could be caused by sleeping on my side and I am a slouch-a-holic.	I will establish healthy sleep-ing habits and positions, good balanced posture, and try to achieve healthy, relatively pain-free muscles.	I will sleep on my back. I will problem solve all the potential hurtful habits contributing to trigger points in these muscles. I will use back supports and place sticky notes to remind me to correct my various standing, sitting, and lying postures. After ruling out concerns with my physician, I will work with a physical therapist to custom design an exercise program.
I have lots of muscle pain, don't sleep well, and have a history of metabolic and nutritional deficiencies similar to those listed in this chapter.	I will decrease muscle pain through the use of proper posture and muscle exercises; increase healthy quality and quantity of sleep, and establish normal metabolic and nutritional levels.	I will establish healthy sleep habits, per Chapter 4. I will schedule my annual checkup and discuss with my doctor my metabolic and nutritional concerns.

9

Step 7: Care for Your Disks and Ligamentous Structures

Let's start with a quick review of the anatomy of the disks and ligamentous structures in your TMJs (see Figure 9.1 on page 171). Your jaw joints each have an articular disk made of a fibrous type of pad that is firm and flexible and shaped somewhat like a donut, with a depression instead of a hole. This disk helps support, protect, and stabilize the joint. Although the disk in your jaw is similar to the cartilage separating the bones in your knees, the disk in your jaw is much more active and dynamic. It is attached by ligaments, a capsule, and tissues, and it moves independently of the bones. The disk is like a moving shock absorber that helps stabilize, separate, and protect the bones above and below from rubbing together.

When you think about it, your lower jaw or mandible is a loose bone that depends on a lot of structures to hold it in place. Ligaments limit movement and soft tissue structures help hold together and stabilize the jaw joint, a bit like ropes or pulleys. Your TMJ has several ligaments, bands, and connective structures; however, for simplification in this chapter, we will primarily focus on the band in the front and back of the joint. In the front, the anterior band attaches the disk to the capsule, where the superior head of the lateral pterygoid also attaches.[1] At the back of the jaw joint in a vascular area referred to as the *bilaminar zone* is the posterior band with an upper and lower part called the *superior and inferior retrodiscal lamina.*

As you open your mouth, the mandible rolls and then glides forward. The disk moves as well, and the posterior band helps stop the disk from moving too far forward. What if these structures are loose or damaged? For your jaws, really loose or damaged structures can make it difficult or impossible for them to do their job of keeping the disk in place. We will talk about this problem more extensively in the second part of this chapter.

Cartilage and joint surfaces generally wear down as we age and cartilage can even disintegrate altogether. This can lead to joint problems and degeneration of the bones. Although the cartilage lining the bones of your TMJ has some ability to heal, uneven wear and bone spurs can develop that sound like crunchy gravel when you open and close your mouth, and these sounds are often a sign that your jaw joint surfaces are wearing down. Excess loading or strain on the ligaments can cause them to fail. According to Rocabado and Iglarsh, ligament failure can lead to a displaced joint and damage to the surrounding structures.[2] In this chapter, we will discuss ways we unwittingly load and strain our ligamentous structures and joints, and how to eliminate these hurtful habits.

Disks

Normally, when you open your mouth, your mandible swings or rotates like a hinge and then glides or translates forward (see Figure 9.1). The disk moves between the top of the mandibular condyle and the temporal bones, preventing them from rubbing together. Several ligamentous type structures help to control the movement of the disk. Among these are the *anterior band* and the superior head of the lateral pterygoid in the front and the *posterior band* in the back of the disk, called the *superior retrodiscal lamina*. These ligamentous structures, which we will refer to as the posterior band, attach the disk to the temporal bone at the back of the joint and act like a leash to help control the forward movement of the disk.[3]

Disk Displacement or Dislocation

Your jaw joint is perhaps the most complex joint in your body, in large part because the disk in your jaw moves. This adds another level

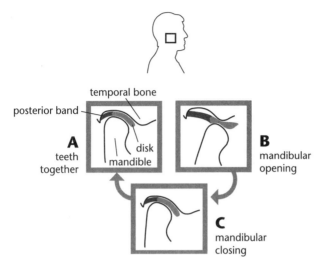

FIGURE 9.1: Normal TMJ disk movement,
opening and closing the mouth

of complexity and also more potential for things to go wrong. Unfortunately, disks can sometimes go astray, often causing pain and dysfunction. The next section of this chapter will discuss some of the primary types of disk displacement and some of the most common causes.

When your teeth are touching your disk should be sitting on top of your mandibular condyle, close to the 12 o'clock position. If the disk is not where it is supposed to be while at rest or during normal movement, this condition is called a *displaced,* or *dislocated, disk.* The disk can displace in many directions, but the most common form of disk displacement is too far forward (anterior) and inside (medial) (see Figure 9.2 on the next page). When a dislocated disk moves back into its proper place, it is referred to as *reduction.* If a dislocated disk fails to reduce, it stays displaced and can cause your jaw to lock.

When a disk is displaced, it does not function properly and will not fully protect the temporal and mandibular bones or function as it was designed to do. A displaced disk that moves in and out of place can also cause clicking, pain, and problems in many of your surrounding muscles and structures. A study by Swedish professor Annika Isberg (with Widmalm and Ivarsson) showed that when the

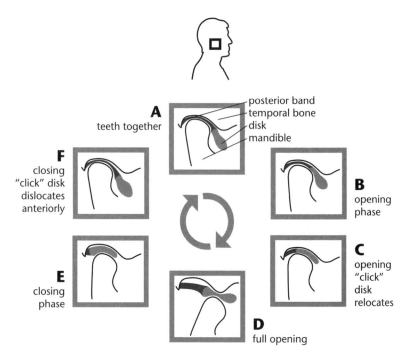

FIGURE 9.2: Anterior disk dislocation with reduction (reciprocal click) when opening and closing the mouth

disk was displaced, the surrounding muscles were highly irritated, but they relaxed back to normal when the disk was put back into place.[4]

Clicking

According to the National Institutes of Health, jaw clicking is fairly common in the general population.[5] In fact, approximately 50 percent of people, without any symptoms, report some TMJ sounds and their lower jaw deviates when they open.[6] However, Rocabado and Iglarsh state, "Because the temporomandibular joint is a friction-free joint, any joint sound should alert the clinician [or make you aware of the possibility] that the synovial joint is malfunctioning."[7] Personally, if I had TMJ sounds or deviation, I would take that as an early warning sign and be motivated to read this book and replace hurtful habits with healthy ones.

Sometimes a loud sound can be heard as you open your mouth. I have had patients who think this is pretty cool and want to do it over and over again. Don't! Rocabado and Iglarsh classify this sequence of events as *high-velocity trauma* to your joints and report it is caused by abnormal alignment of the joint. They put whiplash injuries in the same category and say if the abnormal alignment of the TMJ is not resolved, it will eventually cause joint disease.[8]

The most common jaw sound that can be associated with the disk are clicks, which can be hard to hear without special equipment. The most common cause of a click is an anteriorly displaced disk with reduction. This means the disk is displaced forward, or in front, of the condyle, while at rest. If it is a reciprocal click, an opening click occurs when the disk moves back on top of the condyle as the mouth opens. This is sometimes referred to as an *anterior disk displacement with reduction* because the disk starts in an anterior position in front of the condyle but goes back into place during opening. A closing click occurs when the disk slides forward off the condyle as the mouth closes. Sometimes the clicks are hard to hear (see Figure 9.2). Generally, the later in opening you hear the click, the more concerning your joint situation is and the closer your joint may be to locking.

Locking

There are several reasons for a jaw to lock. The most common cause is an *anteriorly displaced disk without reduction*. This means the disk stays too far in front of the condyle and doesn't slip back into place as it did in the clicking example. As represented in Figure 9.3 on the next page, the disk is forced forward, or anterior, to the mandibular condyle. As this person tries to open his or her mouth, the disk gets in the way. This prevents the mouth from opening all the way. It is common for someone to have lots of pain and clicking in their TMJ, then suddenly the clicking stops and there may even be little or no pain, but their motion is limited. This can be an indication that their jaw has locked, and this condition should be evaluated as soon as possible. According to Kraus, side-to-side movement of the jaw may recapture the disk if it is displaced.[9] However, you should consult with a TMJ expert as soon as possible if you feel that your jaw is locked.

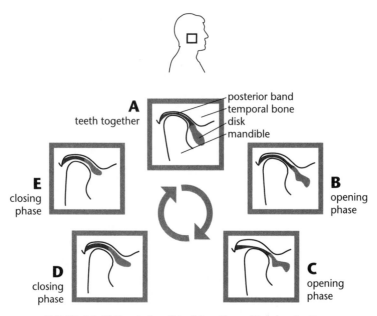

FIGURE 9.3: TMJ anterior disk dislocation without reduction (lock) when opening and closing the mouth

Some people eventually obtain full motion while the disk is still displaced. However, this is not the solution we want. It stretches and damages the posterior band. And even worse, without the protection of the disk between the two bones, the attaching bands and joint surfaces can wear down. This eventually will lead to a chronic TMJ disorder (see Table 9.1). So do not force your jaw to open if there is a chance that it is locked. A locked jaw that won't unlock may require surgery.

Too often there is a progression of symptoms, starting with joint tenderness, leading to occasional clicking and then continual clicking, and finally leading to an acute, or sudden, lock. If the joint stays locked for a long time, joint tissues and structures can be damaged, and it may eventually lead to degenerative arthritis (see Table 9.1).

Overopening the Jaw

Although some people with TMJ disorders need to increase their ability to open their mouth, it is my experience that more need to appropriately limit their opening. How far should you open your

Table 9.1: An All-Too-Common Progression[10]

Level 1	Disk is slightly forward (anterior) and inside (medial), compared to where it should normally rest on top of the mandibular condyle Occasional click (may or may not be present) Mild or no pain
Level 2	Disk is forward (anterior) and inside (medial) There is a click, experienced early on opening and late on closing Severe consistent pain
Level 3	There is a click later on opening and earlier on closing Most painful stage
Level 4	There is rarely a click because the disk no longer moves back into place No pain

mouth? According to the American Academy of Orofacial Pain, you should limit your jaw opening (yawning, etc.) to no more than two fingers' width.[11] Generally, two fingers of your nondominant hand represents approximately 70 to 80 percent of your optimal opening and posterior band length, whereas opening to a width of three fingers elongates the posterior band to almost 100 percent of its length. Anything beyond that is considered overopening and can cause these ligamentous structures that hold the disk in place to become damaged and fail, which can result in disk displacement. You should not regularly open your jaw more than two fingers except when doing exercises prescribed by a TMJ expert.

A young man I knew in college could put his entire fist into his mouth. It was unbelievable. As I have learned more about the jaw and the problems caused from overopening, I have thought of him and hope for the sake of his jaw that he no longer entertains in this manner.

If you prefer not to put your hands into your mouth, you can use what I call the "Rule of Tongue" instead. When you yawn or open wide, keep the tip of your tongue on the roof of your mouth. This gives you a guideline to prevent yourself from opening too wide, without needing to stick your hands into your mouth to measure the extent of opening.

The following are some reasons we tend to overopen and ways to alleviate the problem:

- When **yawning**, keep your tongue on the roof of your mouth to stop you from opening too far. You can also try placing your hand under your chin as you yawn to tell you when to stop.

- Stop **yelling**. Clap, whistle, or make a sign instead of yelling to cheer someone on.

- Avoid **biting into big food**, like big burgers. Try making them smaller by cutting them up or eating the top, then the bottom halves, and chew carefully.

- Tell your **dentist** about your jaw problems, your concern about overopening, and your need to take frequent breaks in the dentist's chair to prevent extended opening of your mouth. Avoid long dental procedures. When necessary, break the procedure up into multiple appointments. Most dentists will be very accommodating. When pressure is being applied to the bottom teeth, place your hand under your chin to help protect the muscles and ligaments of the jaw from becoming overloaded.

- Tell the **anesthesiologist** before any surgery that you have jaw problems. If you are to be unconscious during surgery, the staff will usually pull on your jaw and then intubate (put a large tube down your throat) to keep your airway open during surgery. This could irritate your jaw and force your jaw open for prolonged periods. People who have had multiple surgeries may be more at risk for jaw problems.

- **Intimacies**, such as certain kinds of kissing and oral sex, can put tremendous stress on the jaw joints and muscles. Explain this to your partner and work things out accordingly.

- **Snorkeling and scuba diving** can force your jaw to remain open for extended periods.

- **Vomiting** is not the easiest activity on your jaw. While most vomiting cannot be avoided, bulimics and women who are sick during pregnancy are particularly at risk for jaw problems. Get help if you are bulimic, and talk to your doctor about antinausea measures during pregnancy.

Other Disk Dysfunctions

Disk problems can be caused by more than mere disk displacement. The disk can be displaced, distorted, damaged, and torn by trauma and abnormal loads, which can lead to wear and tear. Without the cushioning and protection the disk provides, the surfaces of the bones can change from being smooth to bumpy and worn down. These bony changes are referred to as *degeneration* or *osteoarthritis*. Physical therapy, splints, and surgery, as well as the healthy habits suggested in this book, are just a few of the tools that can help restore the disk to its proper place and help stabilize its function.

You need to remember that even if the disk is restored to its proper place and function, it is easy for everything else to continue to "limp," or malfunction. Certain muscles and structures may be out of balance and habituated to do things the wrong way. Remember, if you have limped for years because of a hip problem and then have your hip fixed surgically, you may still limp, even though the joint problem is no longer there. You might have to relearn how to walk without a limp. The same can be true for jaw problems. Most of the people I treat with head, neck, and jaw problems cannot open their jaws straight and have to relearn how to use their jaw in a balanced, smooth, and fully aligned way. It is important that the muscles of the jaw work in a coordinated fashion so that all of the associated structures function appropriately.

What You Can Do to Improve Disk Function

Trauma or prolonged pressure to the joint, like sleeping on your stomach, can damage the disks in your jaw. However, healthy, balanced movement is critical for healthy joints and disks. But how do you know if your joint is balanced? One of the ways to check if your joint and muscles are balanced is by watching yourself in a mirror as you open and close your jaw. A normal balanced jaw will usually open and close in a vertically straight manner.

If you have jaw joint problems or muscle imbalances, your jaw may deviate to one side or open with a wiggle or curve. If it does, you can help reeducate your muscles by using the orbiting exercise in the mirror I first discussed in Chapter 5. It is important to do the orbiting exercise in the pain-free and click-free range. Keep in mind that a dislocated disk, tight capsule, or dysfunction of the joint can also cause your jaw to deviate in opening. If there is pain, difficulty, or a chance your jaw joint may be locked, check with your TMJ expert as soon as possible and do not try to push the opening of your jaw.

EXERCISE \ *Orbiting*

With the front third of your tongue on "the spot," slowly open and close your mouth six times (see Figure 5.1 on page 78). Quality, not quantity, of movement is important, so it is best to do this exercise slowly, watching closely in a mirror to ensure you are opening and closing in a manner that is vertically straight. If no mirror is available, you can palpate both joints just in front of your ear. As you open slowly, feel for even and equal rotation on both sides. This is extremely difficult to judge, however, so opt for a mirror if you can. You may want to note a starting point on your teeth to follow to ensure you open straight. Do this exercise six times a day. One easy way to remember is to do it every time you wash your hands during the day, as there is often a mirror available when you do so. However, watch your posture and do not lean into the mirror.

As you work to improve your disk function, your goals should be to keep your disks in their proper place and keep the joint healthy, so you might not have to go on a soft-food diet when you are older. Keep in mind that there are several possible factors affecting this scenario:

- If a portion of the superior head of the lateral pterygoid muscle attaches to the front of the disk and it goes into spasm or is tight, it may pull the disk forward. Muscle spasm and imbalances can affect joint function and how you bite. Splints and physical therapy are often used to help the muscles to relax.

- The posterior band and joint structures may be overstretched due to yawning, whiplash injuries, or macro or micro trauma, or your joints may naturally be overly loose. You may benefit from stabilization exercises.

- Poor posture, a leg-length discrepancy, and rounded shoulders may affect the posture and position of the jaw and abnormally pull on other muscles.

- Psychological and physical stress may activate trigger points and muscle tightness, which can adversely pull on and compress your jaw joints.

All these factors, and others, could be contributing, and each should be addressed for long-term benefits.

Joints, Ligaments, and Hypermobility

Bands, ligaments, the joint capsule, and other connective tissues help stabilize joints, including the jaw joints, by holding them together and controlling their movements. Normal ligaments and tissues are taut and restrict motion, giving joints stability. When these connective tissues are damaged by trauma, both big and small or are naturally loose or lax, you can have *hypermobile* joints. By this term, we mean they move easily beyond their normal range. When this happens, the muscles around the joint must often work harder to help compensate, and the excessive movement can cause more wear and tear on the joints. The joint can become unstable. This is often the case in people with TMJ. Hypermobility also adversely affects the position of the disk. A recent study by German dentist and professor Christian Hirsch (with John and Stang) demonstrated that people with four or more hypermobile joints had a higher risk for reproducible reciprocal clicking in the jaw joints, which can indicate the disk is displaced but reduces or goes back into place during movement.[12]

Excessive joint laxity can lead to wear and tear on joint surfaces and can strain or fatigue the surrounding soft tissue. There are also studies that suggest that people who are hypermobile have impaired sensory feedback from the affected joints, which can lead to excessive joint trauma.[13]

You can have one loose joint or many loose joints. It is common to acquire loose joints in the cervical spine and jaw due to a traumatic event such as a whiplash injury, or hypermobility may occur in joints you frequently stretch or abuse. For example, just as a gymnast who stretches his or her hip joints when doing splits likely has loose hip joints, your jaw joints may be loose from frequent overopening when you yawn or sing, or if you have had multiple surgeries. The joints that are often easiest to recognize as hypermobile are the elbows, wrists, fingers, and knees. However, the TMJ is often involved. Keep in mind that many loose joints throughout the body may be a sign of a syndrome or inherited disorder, including Ehlers-Danlos syndrome, Marfan syndrome, osteogenesis imperfecta, or benign joint hypermobility syndrome.[14]

Hypermobility is often hereditary and is more common in women than in men. Female hormones can make a woman's joints and ligaments more relaxed, particularly when she is pregnant or just before menstruation. People with hypermobile joints often refer to themselves as "double jointed," but how can you know?

Are Your Joints too Loose?

You may have one joint that is too loose, but it is more concerning if most of the joints in your body are loose. But how can you tell? According to the Arthritis Research Commission (ARC), one way to determine if you are generally hypermobile is to try the five movements listed below, which are referred to in the literature as "Beighton's modification of the Carter and Wilkinson scoring system" (now that's a tongue-twister) (see Figure 9.4):[15]

1. Can you bend your thumb back onto the front of your forearm (see Figure 9.4b)?

   Give yourself one point for each thumb you can bend to your forearm or zero points if neither can touch.

2. Can you bend your elbow backward (see Figure 9.4c)?

   Give yourself a point for each elbow that bends backward.

3. Can you bend either of your knees backward (see Figure 9.4d)?

   You get a point for each knee that bends backward.

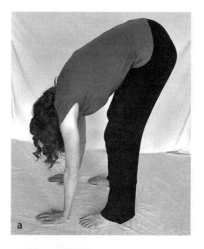

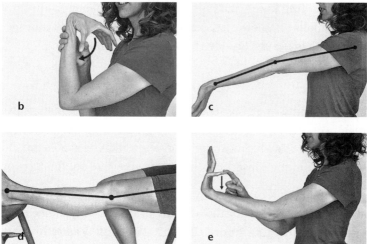

FIGURE 9.4: Joint hypermobility

4. Can you bend your little finger up at 90 degrees (right angles) to the back of your hand (see Figure 9.4e)?

   Give yourself a point for each little finger that can form a right angle.

5. Can you put your hands flat on the floor while holding your knees straight (see Figure 9.4a)?

   If so, give yourself one point.

The maximum score you can get is a 9 on this modified scale. According to The Hypermobility Syndrome Association, a score between 4 and 9 is an indicator that you have widespread hypermobility.[16]

If you answered yes to any of the five questions presented above, you may be at risk for overly loose joints that affect your jaw as well as other joints in your body. If most of your joints are loose, you should talk to your health-care provider to rule out associated disorders and discuss a stabilization program, if appropriate.

What You Can Do to Help Stabilize Your Joints

Research funded by the ARC has shown the value of exercise to strengthen and condition the muscles around your joints. These include your feet, knees, and hips, as they all affect your posture and your jaw joints.[17] These exercises need to be customized to your specific health issues and are not within the scope of this book.

Summary

Your jaw joints, or TMJs, are extremely complex joints that involve many working parts. You should now have a basic understanding of what the disks and ligamentous bands and structures should do, and what some of the consequences are when they are not functioning correctly.

1. It is important that the disks, bands, ligaments, and connective tissues supporting the disks and joints are healthy and structurally sound.

2. Hypermobile joints can make the TMJ unstable and prone to problems.

3. Traumatic, frequent, or lengthy opening of the mouth can damage the joint structures

4. Make yourself a checklist for change. Table 9.2 contains hypothetical examples.

Table 9.2: Checklist for Change: Care for Your Disks and Ligaments

HURTFUL HABIT	HEALTHY HABIT	CHECKLIST FOR CHANGE
I have pain and hear a snapping sound when I open my mouth really wide like yawning or chewing large sandwiches.	I will try and limit opening my mouth to no more than the width of two fingers on my nondominant hand and will stop snapping or popping my jaw.	I will place a finger under my chin when yawning. I will practice opening my mouth in a straight manner, using orbiting exercises in the pain-free, click-free range. I will make my food smaller and cut or divide large foods.
My jaw locks every time I wake up on my stomach.	I will sleep on my back or side. With the help of a specialist I will determine the causes of my jaw locking and investigate all my options.	I will sew a ball into the front of my pajamas to prevent me from sleeping on my stomach. I will schedule an appointment with a TMJ expert to decide my course of action. I will establish the healthy PoTSB TLC habits presented in this book.
I think of myself as "double jointed" and can do all five of the hypermobile movements, based on the Beighton's modification chart in this chapter.	I want to increase the stability of my joints.	I will make an appointment with my doctor to rule out any concerning causes and ask about seeing a physical therapist for a joint protection and stabilization program.

10

Step 8: Halt Head and Neck Pain

Let me tell you about a patient whom we will call Hannah.

Hannah: No More Headaches

Hannah was a smart, white-collar professional who had terrible headaches daily. Her headaches made it difficult for her to drive and function. She tried many treatments and medications and was finally referred to a regional headache center where they did a two-hour consultation and ordered lots of tests, including complete blood, hormone, and allergy testing, sonograms, and a sleep study. The tests showed that some food allergies could be triggering Hannah's headaches, so she was asked to keep a symptom diary to identify those foods. Then she eliminated problematic foods from her diet. However, this treatment didn't entirely solve her problems. She was still having headaches daily and was referred back to physical therapy for evaluation and treatment.

Hannah was referred to me by another physical therapist who had treated her with little success. The therapist demonstrated that Hannah's neck muscles were tight, and he was able to improve the range of motion for her neck, but he did not assess her jaw or the hurtful habits that we've discussed in this book.

My evaluation revealed that Hannah had a tongue thrust

and swallowed incorrectly. She had tight pectoralis muscles and a forward head posture. She slept on her stomach, carried a very heavy purse around all day, and had a hurtful computer and mouse arrangement. We addressed all of these areas, including the tight muscle and fascia, and I introduced her to the concepts in this book.

Hannah did everything she was asked, including addressing her hurtful postures in sitting, standing, and sleeping, and treating her myofascial trigger points. Within three visits she felt 50 percent improved and her headaches had decreased from once per day to once per week. Then I helped Hannah add a cardiovascular program, and we continued problem solving together, which involved changing her computer screen at work, the way she corrected papers, and adjusting the angle of her TV, which she watched at an odd angle. After four more visits, she felt 75 percent improved. I then introduced a strengthening and stabilization program. After eleven visits, she was able to go twenty-seven days without a headache and was successfully discharged on a self-management program.

Nearly everyone has had a headache at some point in their lives, but for some people, headaches are frequent and debilitating. Most people we see in the clinic who suffer from headaches, neck pain, or both also have problems associated with the jaw and the muscles involved in chewing. This chapter looks at these interrelated issues and ways you can rid yourself of them.

Headaches

According to the National Institute of Neurological Disorders and Stroke, over 45 million Americans suffer from chronic, recurring headaches.[1] Approximately 90 percent of all headaches are classified as tension-type headaches, which are caused by tightness in the muscles in your head, neck, jaw, and/or shoulders.[2] Some other types of headaches include migraine headaches and cluster headaches.

What Can Trigger Your Headache?
Finding the cause of your headache is essential if you want to achieve long-term relief.[3] Once you have ruled out those rare but serious

causes, it usually boils down to a combination of triggers that seem to pile up until the proverbial straw breaks the camel's back. Tension headaches are the most common type of headache and are caused by tightness in the muscles in your head, neck, jaw, and/or shoulders. So what makes your muscles tight and irritable? Well, it is important for you to review all the muscles that cause headaches that are detailed in Chapter 8 and come up with lists of ideas for corrections that will eliminate many of the contributing factors to your headaches; however, there are other things that trigger headaches as well. Since headaches are a common symptom of people with TMJ, I would like you to be aware of some of the triggers, or contributing factors. There are hundreds of possible triggers, but here are a few:

- muscular tension, irritability, and stress
- psychosocial and emotional stress
- hurtful postures, asymmetries, or positions (e.g., slouching, sleeping on stomach, carrying heavy purse or brief case, holding phone to ear, using a shoulder grasp)
- not enough sleep, insomnia, unusual sleep patterns
- alcoholic beverages
- dehydration, hunger, and/or missing meals, especially breakfast
- cigarette smoke
- chemical-induced headaches caused by hangovers, paint fumes, fragrances or perfumes, cleaning products, pesticides, etc.
- hormone fluctuation common during a woman's cycle and hormonal changes such as menopause
- a result of crying [4]
- bright or fluorescent lights, flickering lights, sun glare or glare on the computer or TV (if this is a problem have some sunglasses handy)
- sinus congestion or pressure
- nerve irritation (sometimes caused by poor posture)
- some medications that can directly cause headaches or indirectly cause you to clench your teeth, resulting in headaches

- sudden changes in the weather
- jet lag or other issues related to time-zone changes
- tumors or pathologic anomalies
- foods such as chocolate, aged cheese, nuts, wine, and alcohol
- ingredients like caffeine, nitrites and nitrates, MSG, and aspartame
- rebound headaches, which can occur from taking pills for headaches more than two times per week

Tyramine, which is present in varying amounts in most foods and increases as the food ages, is a common cause of headaches and food allergies as well. The National Headache Association has a complete listing for a low-tyramine diet at www.headache.org and provides information that can help you identify foods that potentially trigger your headaches.[5]

Seek a Professional Evaluation

Although headaches with a serious cause are rare, I still advise seeing a physician or headache specialist about your head pain to rule out any serious problems. According to the National Institutes of Health, you should have an immediate evaluation if you have any of the following symptoms:[6]

- sudden, severe headache that is explosive or your "worst ever"
- headache following a blow to your head
- headache that becomes progressively worse over a twenty-four–hour period
- severe headache localized to one eye that has some redness
- headache accompanied by a fever, stiff neck, vomiting, or nausea, numbness, paralysis, disorientation, memory loss, change in vision, or slurred speech
- headaches that recently began to occur, and you are over age fifty, especially if you have impaired vision and pain while chewing

I would also be concerned if it is the first time you have had a headache, or if it was more intense or a different kind of a headache than you typically have experienced and interferes with your daily activities.

Helpful Tools and Treatments

When people get a headache, many think first—and only—of popping a pill to stop the pain. While this may be useful first aid and may work in the short term, by itself it is not a good long-term solution. Pain killers have their place, but do not address the causes of the headache, and pain medications tend to have undesirable side effects, especially if used long term. You can do more than just pop a pill. I'd like to encourage you to become an active participant when it comes to overcoming your headaches. Talk to your health-care providers and educate yourself about the options available. A recent study found that patients whose treatment included a class specifically designed to inform them about headache types, triggers, and treatment options did better than those without.[7] This book provides you with some of that information.

Keep a Symptom Diary

A headache diary is probably the most helpful tool for you to use to track what triggers your headaches or associated symptoms, and a diary can help with controlling them in the future. You may want to create a chart for yourself, like the one presented in Table 10.1. You can also download a symptom diary from our website at www.tmj healingplan.com. Write down and describe when each headache or symptom occurred and its characteristics. Describe any connection to diet, environment, and other situations.

After entering the *date* and *times*, record any warnings or *preceding symptoms* you might have had that your headache or symptoms were coming. Then describe the *intensity* on a 1–10 scale, where 1 is almost nothing and 10 is the worst you can imagine. *Triggers* may include what you ate, how much sleep you got, and stressful activities you engaged in. Then describe the *location* and *quality* of your symptoms. Was the headache throbbing or dull? Did you feel dizzy or did your jaw lock? Once your symptoms improved, did they go away completely, or did they linger? Rate your *relief* on a 1–10 scale.

Table 10.1: Symptom Diary

DATE	START TIME	END TIME	INTENSITY: 1–10	PRECEDING SYMPTOMS	TRIGGERS	LOCATION & DESCRIPTION	RELIEF: 1–10	COMMENTS

Comments can include any other information you feel might be helpful, such as what gave you relief.

You will often start to see patterns. For example, you may notice you always get a headache and neck pain after talking to Aunt Bertha on the telephone. Does she make you stressed out or are you holding the telephone incorrectly when you talk to her? To answer that question, notice if you get a headache when you go to her house or if you get a headache while talking to your best friend on the telephone for an hour—any situation that could help to explain the cause/nature of the headache.

Bring your symptom diary to appointments with your healthcare provider so they can help you interpret your findings and eliminate potential culprits.

Nondrug Treatment Ideas

In addition to keeping a diary to identify and eliminate triggers and contributing factors, here are some other treatment ideas that do not involve drugs.

First aid for headaches. I have had great success using a soft, reusable icepack. Cover it with a cloth and place it at the base of the skull. This is usually magical in alleviating headaches that originate at the base of the skull and radiate around to the sides and front of the head, like an occipital neuralgia. If possible, I often try applying moist heat at the same time to the upper back and moist heat on one side of the face, with ice on the other side. I would then alternate the heat and cold on the jaws every five minutes. Details and precautions will be discussed later in this chapter.

Treat your muscles. Many muscles can cause headache-type symptoms. Review Table 8.1 (on page 132) to determine where your symptoms are located and identify which muscles are the most likely culprits. Be sure to get enough quality sleep. Avoid problematic postures, take breaks, and incorporate healthy movement, stretching, and exercise. There are many fabulous manual techniques and modalities especially helpful for headache patients who need help restoring balance and symmetry and decreasing pain and inflammation that trained professionals can provide.

Change your diet. Diet can sometimes be a cause or contributing factor for headaches. You may have food allergies about which you are unaware. As I mentioned, a symptom diary can be used to identify these foods. It also can be used to rule out foods you might think are triggering your headaches. With your doctor's approval, try eliminating specific foods and additives you think may be culprits. Don't eat these foods for two to four weeks, and see if your symptoms improve. Then add back these foods one at a time and monitor for any headaches or aggravating symptoms. Once you have a good idea of which, if any, foods seem to be causing or aggravating your headaches or discomfort, you can avoid them on a more permanent basis. Visit my website, www.tmjhealingplan.org, for a link to the "headache diet," which lists foods that are common headache triggers.

Neck Pain

Your neck is pretty important, isn't it? It holds up your head, protects your spinal cord and your breathing and eating tubes, and can rotate and pivot in almost any direction. In fact, up to 70 percent of us complain of neck pain each year.[8] It is my experience that most people with TMJ disorders have some degree of neck involvement.

Head, neck, and jaw pain are often related. The muscles and connective tissue in your jaw attach to the head and neck, and these areas attach to your upper back and shoulders. The pain from these structures can extend beyond your head, neck, and jaw and into your arms and fingers and can last for months and often reoccur.

Seek a Professional Evaluation

If you have neck pain, you should see a doctor. You should be seen right away if you have symptoms such as any of the following:

- **Trauma.** Injuries should be examined to rule out any fractures or complications.

- **Tingling, numbness, or weakness.** These sensations, moving down your arm or into your fingers, indicate nerve involvement.

- **Signs of meningitis.** Symptoms such as fever, headache, nausea, or vomiting are causes for concern.

What You Can Do to Alleviate Neck Pain

If you want to get better and stay better, you need to find and treat the causes of your symptoms. I have found that my patients with neck pain have most of the same hurtful habits addressed throughout this book. Treatments for neck pain include most of the same treatments used for the jaw. They very often go together, but most people with neck pain don't realize the strong correlation.

You will notice that many of the trigger point management techniques, including pressure release, massage, stretching, and movement, are actually directed at the neck. You would be wise to review Chapter 8 and problem solve what hurtful habits can be eliminated to improve your neck pain. You can also discuss the exercises and stretches discussed in this book with your health-care provider to determine what type of exercise and stretching program is right for you. However, there are a few treatments for the neck that are not usually used for the jaw, such as cervical mobilization and traction.

You may wake up on your stomach with your head in an awkward position, pull a muscle, or suffer a fall that jolts your neck. These are only a few examples of how your neck or cervical spine can get out of alignment. While there are many methods of restoring alignment, if you have loose joints to start with, it is important to start with the most gentle technique possible to get things realigned, which may include restoring muscle balance first, which allows the joint to re-claim its natural position. Add more direct techniques as needed.

Manual techniques are frequently used on the cervical spine to help relax muscles, unload the joints, and improve the alignment and balance of the neck structures that are integrally connected to the jaw. Often, misalignment of the structures below, such as the pelvis, sets the stage for imbalances in the head and neck above. However, avoid high-velocity thrusts or manipulations that force the joints past their normal range of motion. Also, be aware that sometimes, though very rarely, these aggressive types of movements can increase the risk of stroke, as they can dislodge a clot from the vessels in the neck.[9] It happened to a young mother I knew. Cervical traction is sometimes prescribed and can be beneficial, but it should never put pressure on the jaw joint. Typically, I have a patient lie on his or her back on the table, and I apply manual traction by gently pulling on the base of the skull.

First Aid When You Need It

The first-aid techniques discussed here are for nonemergency times when you overdo or find your head, neck, or jaw irritated or painful. Remember that serious injuries or concerns including dislocation, loss of sensation or strength, or radiating or intense pain always need to be evaluated by a health-care professional.

Cynthia: A Kick in the Jaw

I was helping my four-year-old swing across the monkey bars when one of his arms slipped and he swung his leg in my direc-tion, kicking me in the jaw. I was shocked, but I carefully helped him down. We got into the car, and after assessing that I was just sore, that there was no serious injury, I did a few gentle or-biting exercises in the mirror, while not letting my muscles or joints pull my chin to either side. I kept moving my jaw gently as I drove home, and I applied ice as soon as I could. I made sure I gently moved my jaw muscles throughout the day, icing every couple of hours. I checked my muscles for trigger points and en-sured I was using the healthy habits represented by PoTSB TLC (posture, tongue on the roof, swallowing, breathing correctly and teeth apart, lips together, and calm muscles). I made sure the food I ate was not chewy or painful and that I got a good night's rest. The next day I was a little stiff and kept up my routine, orbiting with a mirror whenever I washed my hands and checking my muscles, and by the third day I felt back to normal.

Decrease Pain and Inflammation

You can use applications of hot, cold, or both to decrease pain and inflammation and to relax muscle spasms. Applying hot or cold packs to the painful area is an inexpensive and effective first-aid technique you can use at home. All you need is an ice pack and/or heating pad and towels. Even the temporary relief of pain and muscle spasm can have long-term benefits because it can break the pain cycle.[10]

Cold

Most people only think of icing immediately after an injury, but it can be helpful even in chronic situations or when heat is not advisable, because heat can increase inflammation.[11] Here are some tips regarding the application of cold:

- Be sure to use a soft, reusable icepack, which can be found at most stores with a pharmacy. You don't want to lie on hard, bumpy ice cubes. I keep my icepacks in the door of the freezer so they do not become too hard. Slip the icepack into a towel or pillowcase and apply to the affected area for 15 to 20 minutes.

- You can also apply cold by rubbing ice cubes or chips along the muscle in the direction of the muscle fibers for not more than seven minutes at a time.[12] I like to gently move or stretch the muscle while I do this.

- If cold irritates a trigger point, switch to moist heat or alternate between cold and heat and repeat as needed.

- Cold can be applied to the base of the skull to help relieve some headaches.

- Ice packs may be used frequently if you have inflamed areas or are in severe pain. However, always be sure that your skin and tissue in the treated area fully return to normal temperature before you reapply ice and to place a pillowcase or towel between you and the ice.

- Do not use ice if you are diabetic, have decreased circulation or sensation in the affected area, have Reynaud's syndrome, peripheral vascular disease, or a "chill stress" sensitivity. Never ice over an open wound.[13] Use caution to avoid frostbite.

Moist Heat

Moist heat can reduce pain, increase circulation, and aid in relaxation. Moist heat is preferable, but dry heat can work as well. Hot showers are a nice form of applying moist heat and a good way to warm up before stretching. Here are some tips regarding the application of heat:

- Heat can be applied in the form of a hot, wet towel or a moist heating pad and usually lasts 15 to 20 minutes.[14]

- Use extreme caution to prevent burns and only use a heating pad that has an automatic shut-off feature.

- Do not use heat if you have impaired circulation, reduced sensation, or hemorrhagic conditions, as well as those precautions listed for cold.

- Use caution when applying heat directly over the temporomandibular joint, because it can sometimes irritate an already inflamed joint.[15] If you need to apply heat to the muscles on the side of your face, you can usually avoid irritating an inflamed joint by placing the heating pad just in front of the joint, which sits in front of your ear. You can also protect the joint from direct heat by using extra towels. Discuss this treatment with your doctor or physical therapist.

Applying Hot and Cold at the Same Time

I often have the best results when I use hot and cold at the same time. Here are some tips regarding the multiple uses of concurrent hot and cold applications:

- You may need to have multiple cold packs and moist heat packs available. If I want to apply ice to the base of my skull, moist heat on my upper back and neck, and alternate hot and cold on my jaws, I will need two cold packs and two moist heat packs of appropriate size.

- I have a lot of success applying moist heat to one side of the face and cold to the other for five minutes. Switch sides every five minutes for a total of 15 to 20 minutes, as tolerated. Try starting and ending by using cold on the side that is swollen or inflamed.

Move Gently in the Pain-Free and Click-Free Range

Gentle movement can help relax the muscles in your jaw and neck and decrease inflammation. Keep your tongue on the roof of the mouth and open and close only in the click-free and pain-free range. Movement of irritated muscles and joints is important in maintaining mobility, pumping fluid in and out of the joint, and helping to prevent muscles from becoming tight or going into spasm.

PoTSB TLC as First Aid

You can use PoTSB TLC for first aid by quickly reviewing these important steps, much as I did in the incident I described in which my child accidently kicked me in the jaw. Just go through them, one by one, and check yourself:

Posture in sleeping, standing, and sitting
Tongue on the roof
Swallow correctly
Breathe well
TLC: Teeth apart, **L**ips together, and **C**alm the muscles and mind

Check Muscles and Treat Trigger Points

You can use the techniques discussed in Chapter 8 as part of your first aid. Find active trigger points and eliminate them by gently releasing and massaging the irritated muscles to increase relaxation and circulation. Use the problem-solving sections for each muscle to identify and eliminate the causes, contributors, and other hurtful habits that may also irritate the muscles. Then gently stretch and move. As always, check with your health-care provider first and discontinue if the exercises increase your pain or dysfunction.

Summary

Now that you know some of the causes of headaches and neck pain, common treatments, and warning signs that should be addressed right away, let's review some of the main points:

1. Most of us experience headaches and neck pain, but few of us take the time or know how to identify and manage common triggers.

2. If you really want to uncover some of the causes of headaches, start a symptom diary.

3. Then, when setbacks occur, you can try some of the first-aid tools to help get you over the hump and quickly back on the road to recovery.

4. Make yourself a checklist for change. Use Table 10.2 as a guide. Remember, these are examples, not treatment recommendations.

Table 10.2: Checklist for Change: Head and Neck

HURTFUL HABIT	HEALTHY HABIT	CHECKLIST FOR CHANGE
I have daily headaches and like to watch television at an angle in my recliner.	I understand and can manage many of the postures that trigger headaches.	I will sit up when watching television and move my chair so the television is not at an angle. I will use pillows or arm supports to unload the weight of my shoulders and arms and decrease the strain on my neck when sitting. I will make a first-aid plan.
I always pop a pill for my head and neck pain and then keep doing what I am doing.	I will be able to improve my head and neck pain with non-drug options as well.	I will try using hot and cold packs and have them on hand to help alleviate my symptoms. I will stop what I am doing and problem solve triggers contributing to my headaches. I will keep a headache diary. I will identify and eliminate trigger points in my muscles.

HURTFUL HABIT	HEALTHY HABIT	CHECKLIST FOR CHANGE
I work on the computer all day and come home with a sore neck and headache every day that seems to start at the back of my head. I wear bifocals.	I will be able to work on the computer without having a headache at the end of the day.	I will ergonomically arrange my computer and workstation and problem solve other areas. I will buy a separate pair of glasses to wear when I am using the computer. I will take microbreaks in the day to move and stretch. I will try ice at the back of my head and moist heat on my neck and shoulders.

11

Step 9: Reduce Stress and Begin to Exercise

You have felt it before. You have a close call and almost trip down the stairs. Your heart starts racing, and your breathing becomes more rapid. This is the fight-or-flight response and it exists to protect you from danger. When you perceive a threat, powerful chemicals and hormones are released that help prepare your body for emergencies. Blood is redirected from your skin and internal organs toward your muscles and brain. Your muscles become tense so that you are ready to flee or fight. Although most of us are seldom in true danger, we too frequently react to day-to-day challenges as if we were. In this chapter, we look at the role stress plays in TMJ disorders and at ways to overcome harmful stress.

Fight-or-Flight Versus Rest-and-Digest

The fight-or-flight response is a reaction initiated by our autonomic nervous system (ANS). Our ANS does things automatically, without our needing to think about them. Breathing and digestion are two examples of automatic processes handled by the ANS. The ANS, which regulates most of the organs and muscles in our body, has two branches that are responsible for opposite kinds of reactions. One branch handles emergencies and causes the fight-or-flight response. The other branch handles nonemergencies. Instead of fight-or-flight, it lets us rest-and-digest.

Some stress is good and is a natural part of everyday life. It can help us learn and grow. Some physical stress can be important, too. For example, the stress you feel when you realize your house is on fire might help you get out quickly, and the stress of weight-bearing is beneficial for people at risk for osteoporosis because it makes their bones stronger. However, prolonged and hurtful stress can adversely affect our posture and breathing, cause us to clench or grind our teeth, and increase the tension in our muscles. This irritates our head, neck, and jaw and can cause pain, which only adds to our stress and can create a vicious cycle.

People who are constantly in pain are also constantly under stress. Emotional stress, as well as physical stresses, such as overly loose joints or multiple trigger points, can overload the nervous system. Some researchers believe the common link between TMJ disorders and a multitude of other chronic pain disorders like fibromyalgia may be that the central nervous system (CNS) is stuck in high gear, resulting in a debilitating cycle of pain and dysfunction.[1] When the nervous system is constantly bombarded, it can lead to oversensitization. You can become hypersensitive to lights, sounds, smells, pain, and so forth. This can be even more aggravating if you are told it is "All in your head," when your suffering is very real.

Tragically, some people suffering from TMJ-related disorders are also victims of physical, sexual, or psychological abuse. This makes it extremely difficult for them to ever feel safe. Because many don't feel safe, their fight-or-flight response may be constantly turned on. In this state, it may be impossible to completely resolve TMJ disorders and the associated symptoms without the appropriate (psychological) help. Many others with TMJ-related disorders suffer from anxiety or depression. People are often hesitant to admit that their stress and emotions have anything to do with their symptoms.[2]

Constant levels of stress can lead to physiological problems, including chronic muscle tension and muscle disorders, such as TMJ disorders, myofascial pain, and fibromyalgia; headaches; difficulty sleeping; gastrointestinal problems, such as irritable bowel disease; heart disease; high blood pressure; a decreased pain tolerance; and the list goes on. Chronic or severe stress can weaken your immune system, overwork your heart, deposit fat at your waist, and damage memory cells. Prolonged or harmful stress can also lead to psychological problems, including anxiety disorders and depression.[3] Of course, physical and psychological stress may not be the singular cause of your head, neck, and jaw pain; however, there is no doubt it can be a significant contributing factor. When taking a patient's history, I have noticed that a patient's onset of symptoms frequently coincides with a stressful event or events. This stressful event may make it more difficult for them to sleep well or exercise, and things can snowball from there. Let me better illustrate this point with an example. I recently had two patients with similar symptoms. They also both had stressful jobs. However, one of them was overwhelmed by a life-changing event (events that fall into this category are job loss, abuse, divorce, and death of a close friend or family member). While one felt 90 percent improved in three visits, the one experiencing the life-changing event reported little or no improvement in the same number of visits.

Even if your pain does not improve as you replace hurtful habits with healthy ones, you are still better off in the long term. If no improvement is made and you are doing everything you are supposed to do, it is usually an indication that there are other contributing factors that need to be explored and addressed, and stress is often the culprit.

Dr. Jon Kabat-Zinn, founding director of the Stress Management Clinic at the University of Massachusetts Medical Center, shares a vivid example of the effects of stress. He saw a fifty-four-year-old woman to help her control her stress to lower her blood pressure. Her medical charts stood over four feet tall. She had several chronic health problems including neck and back pain, heart disease, arthritis, lupus, ulcers, and repeated urinary tract infections, and she was also not sleeping well, staying awake for long periods in the middle of the night. She had endured four years of sexual abuse but was married with five kids. After finishing the stress-management program, which included working through her feelings and emotions, her blood pressure dropped from 165/105 to 110/70, she routinely slept through the night, and her neck and back pain improved.[4]

What You Can Do to Reduce Stress

Unfortunately, even when a stressor or danger is not real, our perception of the situation as a threat can kick our body into a fight-or-flight state of constant tension. Too many of us are stressed, tense, and uptight much of the time. I like to use the analogy that stress is like driving down a really steep hill. If you don't apply your brakes regularly or consciously, or switch to a lower gear, the stress levels can veer out of control. This is why activities such as diaphragmatic breathing, relaxation, meditation, and yoga can be so helpful. When done correctly, they can help apply the brakes by helping our body turn off this unwanted automatic response and return to a more normal and relaxed state. They can move us from fight-and-flight toward rest-and-digest. You must find the stress-management strategies that work best for you and use them when you notice the first signs of stress. The physical therapists I work with at Canyon Rim Physical Therapy are trying some exciting methods that work to successfully calm down the nervous system. Although supportive research is scarce, the initial results are encouraging.

The following is a list of ways you can slow down your escalating stress:

Breathe! Some believe that as few as five slow, relaxed breaths taken through your nose, engaging the diaphragm, can help kick you out of the fight-or-flight response and into the rest-and-digest mode. (See Chapter 7 for more breathing tips and information.)

Sweat and stretch it off. Exercise is a common and beneficial stress reliever. Walk away the stress, do five minutes of Tai Chi, or even do ten jumping jacks followed by a gentle stretch of those tight muscles that will help release the tension and encourage your whole body to relax. You may find that you tend to harbor stress in certain muscles. (More on exercise can be found later in this chapter, and several stretches are discussed in Chapter 8.)

Mind over matter: meditate, visualize and imagine. Meditation and practices such as yoga and Tai Chi, when done correctly, help to focus and calm your mind and body. Our clinic has found much success with meditation and the use of guided imagery. You can listen to a CD or audiotape of the instructions every night before going to sleep. This not only helps you to relax, but it also helps you visualize yourself in healthy, relaxed postures, positions, and habits. It can reinforce all the good habits you are trying to establish and help you calm your muscles and mind at the same time. Go to www.tmjheal ingplan.com for a list of resources we find successful.

Relax and release the tension. Scan your body for tension and then let that tightness melt away. If it is hard for you to tell if you are uptight in certain areas, try the Contract, Relax exercise described on page 118. This will help you locate the areas in which you tend to hold the most tension and to experiment with ways that allow you to relax those areas.

Talk your way out of it. During extremely stressful events, it helps to discuss the traumatic event with someone you trust as soon as possible after the event. This can lessen extreme pathological reactions to stress and may prevent or reduce the development of post-traumatic stress disorder. However, even if it has been years or decades, you can still benefit from working through your feelings and emotions with a person or group who can empathize, understand, and help you move forward in healthy, appropriate ways.

Feel safe and socialize. Establish a safe environment, using familiar music sounds and safe relationships. In *Psychology Today*, neuroscientist Steven Porges says engaging socially with others triggers neural circuits that calm the heart, relax the gut, and switch off fear. Something as simple as a sweet smile, a soothing voice, or gentle eye contact can help you feel safe, so the fight-or-flight stress response can turn off. A good laugh can also do wonders.[4]

Think positively. Negative emotions lead to more pain than positive emotions. Fill your environment with as many positive influences as possible, such as pleasant music, smells, funny movies, and a positive friend. In *Why People Don't Heal, and How They Can*, author Caroline Myss points out that thinking of ourselves as wounded or ill only reinforces poor health. Making an effort to do the opposite and to think positive thoughts not only reduces stress but also promotes physical healing. Visualize yourself as a healthy and happy person involved in healthy activities, postures, and habits.[5]

Understand and overcome your fears. By understanding how fear and other negative emotions adversely affect healing, you may more easily identify how you are interfering, consciously or unconsciously, with your own healing process. You may want to get treatment for phobias or anxiety disorders that are problematic.

Avoid destructive habits. Unfortunately, many of us resort to hurtful habits to cope with stress, such as drugs, pain medicines, alcohol, smoking, and eating. These actually worsen the stress and can make us more sensitive to further stress.

Organize and prioritize. Always get done the things that have to happen to sustain life, but seriously assess the nonessentials and don't overburden or overwhelm yourself. Slow down! Make lists. Eliminate time wasters, but always make time for yourself and your healthy relationships. Allow yourself extra time to get to and from appointments. Being late adds a lot of stress.

Sleep it off. Always get enough rest. Stress is very exhausting, and when we are stressed, we often get even less sleep. Make sure you are getting a good quality of seven to nine hours of sleep per night, depending on what you need to feel well rested.

Keep a journal. Write down your stresses in a journal, and then let them go.

Do a kind deed or gesture. Helping others not only uplifts them, it uplifts you and helps to counteract stress. It is hard to respond using the fight-or-flight response when you are comforting or helping someone else.

Seek professional help. Many people suffering from TMJ-related problems suffer from depression. It is hard to know what came first. Your symptoms are likely not "all in your head," but ignoring your mental health will only make things worse. Just as we need our physical posture to be balanced, we also need our mind and emotions to be balanced. You may be carrying an emotional load that is too heavy and may need someone or a group to help you carry and unload it. Or you may need medication to help balance your hormones and chemicals. We don't think twice about taking calcium if we have osteoporosis, but for some reason we hesitate if we need medication to help balance our minds and emotions. But be sure to do your homework before choosing the right specialist to help you, because just like physical medicine, psychological medicine has speciality areas (e.g., people who have been sexually abused or who are grieving the loss of a family member may benefit most from working with a professional specializing in the field in question and from groups targeted to their specific needs). Please get appropriate help, and remember that there are good and bad doctors in any specialty. As you heal emotionally, you set the stage to heal better physically.

Cynthia: The Stresses of Being an Author

The final writing and compiling of this book came at a tremendously stressful time in my life. We had just moved and had all the firsts that come with a move. For the previous six months, we were living in my in-laws' basement while we waited for our home to sell in Kansas and tried to find a new home during a troubled economy. I have three wonderful and very involved children, and I was working, teaching classes, and writing this book in my "spare time." At times, the stress seemed unbearable. I could tell when the stress was getting out of hand because my muscles would tense and my breathing would become quick and shallow. I knew at those times I had to take immediate action. I would try to relax all my muscles and take several slow, deep breaths until I regained some control. I would do jaw exercises and stretches that lengthened my tightened muscles. I then made time to exercise, talk to a loving friend, or do a kind deed. When I could, I listened to a meditation and guided imagery tape. Once I was so stressed that I tried to listen to tapes while I was driving, which I would not recommend. It also helped to laugh, sometimes cry, and always look for the silver lining that is there if you look hard enough.

Remember, nothing will change unless you do! You have to be committed to eliminating your hurtful habits. Although there are promising treatments for stress, the management of stress is mostly dependent on the willingness of a person to make the changes necessary for a healthy lifestyle. Although some stressors cannot be changed, many are within your control.

Regular Exercise: A Cycle of Success

The U.S. Department of Health and Human Services' *Physical Activity Guidelines for Americans* summary states, "Being physically active is one of the most important steps that Americans of all ages can take to improve their health."[6] Most of us know that exercise is good for us. However, few really understand all of the ways it can benefit us. We might not realize that it is one of the most effective ways to reduce stress as well as improve our overall health.

Everyone can benefit from exercising, including people with disabilities. Let's make a list of some of the benefits of appropriate moderate and vigorous exercise:[7]

- improves the function of your ligaments, joints, and tendons (this means your neck and jaw as well)
- increases blood flow to all organs, including the heart, lungs, and brain
- increases oxygen capacity, energy production, and waste removal
- improves your muscle strength and body composition
- improves your immune system
- improves your mood
- decreases anxiety
- is helpful for weight loss and maintenance
- improves your sleep (but don't exercise close to bedtime)
- raises your self-esteem and sense of well-being
- relieves stress and makes you more resilient to stress
- improves your brain health

- relieves and prevents depression
- improves executive functions, such as ability to focus and select appropriate behaviors
- decreases your likelihood of getting Alzheimer's disease
- releases endorphins that can have an analgesic effect, decreasing your pain
- reduces the risk of many diseases
- improves bone health
- improves thinking ability

The list goes on. Are you motivated to get moving? Any one of the items on this list can serve as your motivation, including the fact that exercise can increase your life expectancy.[8] Your situation does not need to be as dire as that faced by Charles, related below.

Charles: Aerobics after an Accident

Early in my career, I was assigned a 19-year-old named Charles who had been in a serious car accident. He had fractured his neck and lost the strength and feeling in one arm and hand. He was in a halo, which means they put a metal ring that looks like a halo around the top of his head and attach it with screws all around the outside of his head. The contraption is supported by tall metal poles attached to a shoulder harness to stabilize the head so the fracture can heal. He was incredibly motivated and optimistic. We got the doctor's permission to start him on an aerobic exercise program. He slowly worked up to doing an hour or more a day before our treatments and healed much more quickly and fully than doctors anticipated, with a full return of strength and feeling to his arm.

Types of Exercise

There are two main types of exercise: aerobic and anaerobic. Both are useful in reducing stress.

Aerobic Exercise

Aerobic exercise literally means exercise "with oxygen." When you are doing an aerobic exercise, you typically use your larger muscles, which uses up oxygen more quickly. This helps to improve your body's ability to consume oxygen and builds endurance. It helps strengthen your heart and lungs and brings about most of the benefits we have previously discussed. To maximize the benefits of aerobic exercise it should be performed frequently, for example, three to five times per week, and for a sufficient duration of time at the correct intensities, which we will discuss later in this chapter.[9]

Some examples of aerobic exercise are walking, stationary biking, swimming, and using the elliptical trainer. Exercising in warm water is a great way to work out, particularly if you have myofascial pain or painful joints. Moderate exercise is the standard type recommended. However, vigorous exercise near the top of your range is also recommended periodically, provided you are in good enough condition.

Anaerobic Exercise

Exercises that don't require you to use as much oxygen are called *anaerobic*, or "without oxygen." These exercises are performed for shorter durations, but they involve greater intensity. Some anaerobic exercises (e.g., yoga) focus on stretching and increasing flexibility, while others (e.g., weight lifting) focus on strength training and on building muscles and bones.

How Aerobic Exercises Help TMJ Disorders

So what does aerobic exercise have to do with your head, neck, and jaw? Let me explain by telling you about my husband's experience.

Bruce: Dash for the Digit

My husband, Bruce, suffered from what I call "mouse finger." While he was at the computer, his right index finger was in use throughout most of the day, leading to a significant overuse injury. We got a new mouse and tried several exercises, icing, and stretching, with little improvement. After about a year, he decided to start running, and his finger impairment improved 80 to 90 percent.

Who would have thought that running with his legs would make such a significant difference for his finger. How can this be? When you can't exercise a body part directly, you can often get the benefits of exercising by going in through the back door. Suppose you have a broken leg and want the injured leg to obtain the benefits of exercise. With your doctor's permission, you can ride a stationary bike, with your well leg secured in the foot strap, while your broken leg rests on a chair. Even though your broken leg is doing nothing, it still benefits from an overall increase in circulation and your entire body becomes energized. Improved circulation promotes healing and the health of all your muscles and tissues.

My experience is that people who exercise regularly typically get better faster than do sedentary people with the same problem, even if they can't move their affected body part and have to enter the exercise arena by using the back door. People with fibromyalgia, chronic myofascial pain, and other disorders need to approach exercise extremely carefully, as their muscles are typically ultrasensitive and can be easily irritated.

How Much Exercise Is Enough?

The *Physical Activity Guidelines for Americans* put out by the U.S. Department of Health and Human Services provides guidelines for how much and what type of exercise are needed by people of different ages. The guidelines stress aerobic activities, but also include anaerobic exercise.[10]

Children and Adolescents

The guidelines for children at least 6 years old and adolescents are as follows:

- Engage in 1 hour or more of physical activity daily.
- Most of the hour should involve moderate to vigorous aerobic activity.
- Three days a week, the activity should be vigorous and include muscle- and bone-strengthening exercises.
- Exercise should be fun, age appropriate, and varied.

Adults

The guidelines for adults ages 18 through 64 are as follows:

- Be as physically active as possible.

- Engage in 2½ hours of moderate or 75 minutes of vigorous aerobic physical activity, or an equivalent combination of moderate and vigorous intensity aerobic activity.
- Aerobic activity should be in at least 10-minute increments.
- Exercise should be spread throughout the week.
- Exercising for 5 hours a week will produce greater benefits.
- Include muscle-strengthening activities that are moderate or high intensity and involve all major muscle groups on 2 or more days a week.

Older Adults

Adults age 65 and older should follow the adult guidelines, with the following caveats:

- Determine the level of effort based on level of fitness.
- Learn how chronic conditions affect the ability to exercise safely.
- Be as physically active, as abilities and conditions allow.
- Engage in balancing exercises if there is risk of falling.

Start Your Exercise Program

Now you know about the benefits of exercise and the guidelines. But how do you start and which exercises are best? You may think getting up off the couch to walk to the fridge counts as exercise. Sorry! It may be better than nothing, but to get all the benefits, you need to work up to a more vigorous pace.

Safety Recommendations

I recommend you consult with a doctor before beginning an exercise program. Every individual is different and many have multiple health problems. If you have fibromyalgia, stretching may be problematic. If you have heart disease, you need to be watched carefully. I have had several patients with neck or jaw pain and multiple sclerosis, and exercise that increases their core body temperature can make their MS symptoms worse, so to keep them cool, exercises must often be done differently. Although exercise is for virtually everyone, if you have not been exercising for years, you might need to go about it more cautiously. With your doctor's input, pick an exercise that is easy for you to do. In most circumstances, I recommend that you start by doing 2 to 3 minutes of exercise and progress by adding 1 or 2 minutes during each exercise session to determine how well you tolerate it. You may be fine when you get to 20 minutes, but 25 minutes might be too much. If you want to exercise longer, you may need to combine different exercises. Variety is important, and you must listen to your body as you go.

Before you start any exercise program, it is helpful to keep in mind safety precautions. Understand the risks, but be confident that physical activity is safe for almost everyone. Here are some tips:

- Choose exercises appropriate for your current fitness level, underlying conditions, and health goals.

- If you have been leading an inactive lifestyle, "Start low and go slow." Don't try to do too much too fast. Even if you are active, if you haven't done anything for a week or two, start slow. Weekend warriors are common visitors to PT clinics.

- Increase your physical activity gradually over time to meet your goals.

- Protect yourself by using appropriate gear and sports equipment, looking for safe environments, following rules and policies, and making sensible choices about when, where, and how to be active.

- Work with your health-care provider if you have chronic conditions or symptoms, are pregnant or postpartum, or have a disability, in order to make sure you are doing the appropriate types and amounts of activity for you.

- Jarring types of exercise, such as jogging, can be hard on the joints and some muscles, including the jaw and neck.

- Good posture is important even when you exercise. I have been on a treadmill next to people so hunched over that it hurts me to even watch them.

Design an Aerobic Program

The purpose of an aerobic exercise program is to get your heart rate up and to move at an intensity that will benefit your body and reduce stress, but that does not overdo it.

Finding Your Level of Intensity

So how intensely should you exercise? There are several methods you can use to monitor yourself to maximize the benefits you desire. Two methods I recommend are the heart rate method and the perceived exertion scale. Choose the one that works best for you.

The Heart Rate Method. The heart rate method uses the following formula to determine your maximum heart rate (note that this is *not* the target heart rate you should reach while exercising):

220 – Age = Maximum Heart Rate

Then, calculate the target heart rate you want to reach while you exercise; that is, how intensely you want to exercise. This is usually between 50 and 85 percent of your maximum heart rate, depending on your age, fitness level, and goals. So if you are 20 years old, your maximum heart rate would be 200. If you are in great shape, you would multiply the heart rate (200) by 70 to 85 percent (0.7–0.85) which would tell you that while you are exercising, your heart rate should stay between 140 to 170 beats per minute. If you were in poor shape or haven't exercised in a while, you would likely start in the 50 to 70 percent range (0.50–0.70), which would tell you to keep your heart rate between 100 and 154. Table 11.1 gives another example, using a typical 35-year-old.

Table 11.1: Calculating a Target Heart Rate for a 35-Year-Old Working at a 70 Percent Target Heart Rate

FORMULA	EXAMPLE
220 – Age x 0.7 = Target Heart Rate	220 – 35 = 185 x 0.7 = 129.5

How do you take your heart rate while you are exercising? The easy way is to use a machine that takes your pulse for you or wear a heart-rate monitor. The old-fashioned way is a little more complex.

It is easier to feel your pulse if you stop moving. Set the back of your right wrist in the palm of your left hand. Then let the fingers on your left hand wrap around the thumb side of your right wrist. You should feel a pulse. Now find an analog clock with the hands that spin around or set a timer for 15 seconds and count how many beats you get during the 15-second period and multiply that number by four. If you have the patience, you can take your pulse for the full minute. The result will indicate your heart rate, or how many beats per minute your heart is pumping.

Perceived Exertion Scale. Perceived exertion is another method, and it represents how hard you perceive your body to be working. Are you sweating and breathing hard, and is your heart racing? Or are you bored and barely working? This is a subjective, but usually fairly accurate, system. I like to keep it simple, using the following 0–10 scale:

0 = Nothing at all.

1 = Easy as pie sliding off your fork.

2 = Like a slow summer stroll.

3 = You are still comfortable, but breathing a bit harder.

4 = You are starting to sweat but you can talk without being out of breath.

5 = You are starting to have to work, sweating more, but still talking. However, if you were to sing, you would be out of breath.

6 = You can still talk, but even talking is making you out of breath.

7 = Very intense. You don't want to talk anymore and you're dripping with sweat.

8 = So intense you can't keep it up for long.

9 = You would only keep up this pace if you were being chased by a runaway truck.

10 = You feel like you have been run over by the truck.

I might start a sedentary person with chronic pain with one to two minutes in the 1-to-2 range. But for an active person, I would spend more time in the 5-to-6 range and eventually slowly work in some vigorous bouts up into the 7-to-8 range, if tolerated. It is your body and you need to decide, after consultation with your doctor, what is best for you, depending on your health situation and exercise goals. How you begin and end your exercise is very important in preventing injuries, muscle tightness, and soreness. You need to establish a healthy routine.

Set Up a Routine

Remember, you can think of your muscles like bubble gum. You can't blow bubbles with cold gum and you can't safely do all you want with a muscle unless it is warm. When muscles are warm, they are less likely to become injured. So always start your exercise with a warm-up. Usually, this is as simple as starting your activity slowly for five to ten minutes. You know you are warmed up if you start to perspire.

Because you shorten your muscles while doing aerobic exercise, you should return them to their normal length when you are done by stretching (see Table 11.2). I often encourage my patients to do the stretches and exercises I have given them for their head and neck problems after doing their aerobic exercise while their muscles are warm. Warm muscles tend to tolerate the movements better and seem to provide better results.

Table 11.2: A Sample Aerobic Routine

Warm up and optional stretch	Start slowly into your exercise. Once you start to sweat, your muscles are warm. You can now stretch when your muscles are warm.
Exercise	Walking, water walking, swimming, stationary cycling, etc.
Stretch after	Cool down at the end of your exercise and stretch at least the muscle groups used while exercising, as well as those that are tight.

Design a Stretching Program

It is best to cool down and stretch after you've exercised as well. If your muscles are like bubble gum, warm gum will cool and harden in whatever position you leave it. If you leave it on your fork, it will fill in the blanks and cool with the imprint of a fork. The same is somewhat true for muscles. Too often, my patients exercise and then sit in the car and then sit hunched over at their work while their muscles cool and harden into a shortened position of poor posture. This is true for all your muscles, including the muscles in your head, neck, and jaw. Even if you have only exercised your legs, once you start sweating, your body temperature is warm enough that all your muscles will warm up. Take this opportunity to help the muscles to return to healthy lengths and positions.

Stretching should be done slowly in the pain-free normal range of motion. Don't bounce when you stretch. It is okay if you feel a gentle pull but not if you feel pain. If you feel pain, back off as much as you need to in order to stay in the pain-free range.

If you have overly loose joints or sensitive muscles, you must be extremely careful. You likely need a stabilization program more than a stretching one. It would be best to design your exercise program with your physical therapist or health-care provider. For example, when stretching the hamstring muscles in your legs, you need to learn to stop when your knee is straight and not let it buckle backward beyond its normal range. You probably need to stretch for shorter periods, but muscle imbalances might be more of a problem. If you have one side of your jaw that is tighter than the other side, it is very likely that every time you open your mouth, your jaw will deviate toward the tight side.

How Frequently Should You Stretch?

Travell and Simons recommend stretching sore muscles every day gently through their full normal range of motion to ensure continued relief from trigger points.[11] I recommend that my patients do the majority of their stretches after exercising when their muscles are still warm. However, tender, tight muscles may need to be elongated several times a day.

How Long Should You Stretch?

Any stretching or movement can help, but I recommend you hold the stretch about 5 to 10 seconds. For muscles that are tight, you might want to hold the stretch for a total of 30 to 60 seconds. However, I usually break the stretching process into segments; for example, hold the stretch for 10 seconds and repeat it three to six times. Find what works best for you. If you are sore after stretching, you usually did the stretch incorrectly or pulled too hard. It is always better to understretch than to overstretch, in order to avoid injury to a muscle. The next time you stretch after being sore, go half as far as you did the previous time. If you continue to have discomfort, discontinue the stretch and call your therapist. There are several ways to stretch each muscle and some people need a variation. Please check with your health-care provider before including them in your regimen.

Important Stretches

Because most aerobic exercise (e.g., walking) uses your leg muscles, and tight leg muscles can adversely affect your posture, it is important to regularly stretch the hamstrings, quadriceps, and calves, especially after you exercise. I will explain the basics, but you may need a variation depending on your situation.[12]

EXERCISE \ *Hamstring Stretches*

Lying on your back, with your knees straight, lift one leg and wrap your hands under your thigh, just above your knee so your hip and back form a 90 degree angle. Now slowly try to straighten your up knee. You should feel a stretch but no pain. If this is too much stretch you can bend the lower leg to make it easier. Hold for five to ten seconds, then repeat three to six times. Switch legs and repeat the stretching process.

You can also stretch the hamstring muscles while sitting on the floor or side of a bed with one leg stretched out straight in front of you and the other knee bent or rotated outward. Lean forward over the straight leg, bending at the hips and not the waist, while keeping your knee and back straight. If you feel a stretch without even bending forward, you can place an arm behind you for support to help you maintain a gentle stretch (see Figure 11.1 on the next page).

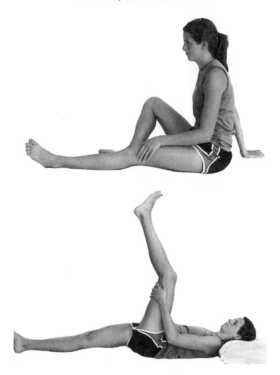

FIGURE 11.1: Ways to stretch the hamstring muscles

> EXERCISE   *Quadriceps Stretch*
>
> You can perform this stretch standing or lying sideways on the bed or floor. Gently pull your foot toward your buttocks using the same-side hand. Keep your hips straight; do not arch your back. Hold the stretch for five to ten seconds and repeat three to six times (see Figure 11.2).

> EXERCISE   *Calf Stretch*
>
> While keeping your heels on the ground, step forward and hold the back knee straight. Hold for five to ten seconds and repeat three to six times. Repeat with the back knee bent (see Figure 11.3).

Design a Strength-Training Program

Strength training can be a touchy subject for people with head, neck, and jaw pain. I usually start strength training last. If a person has sore muscles, my emphasis would be on first eliminating trigger

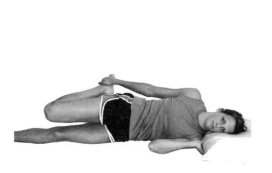
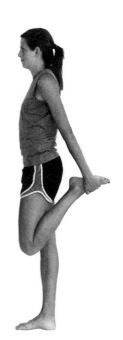

FIGURE 11.2: Ways to stretch the quadriceps muscles

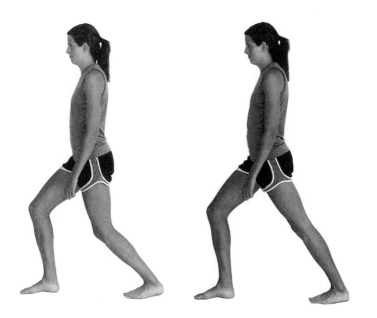

FIGURE 11.3: Ways to stretch the calf muscles

points and regaining the full range of motion through movement and stretching exercises, then starting a smart and gentle program for strength and balance.

Balance is a key word when it comes to strength training. Most of the buff men I see at the gym are out of balance. Their upper-neck and chest muscles are typically too strong, their mid-back muscles are weak, and they have rounded shoulders. Most of the circuit machines encourage this imbalance. Your strengthening efforts should make it easier for you to achieve balanced posture, not make you lopsided. If you strengthen in one direction, you should usually counterbalance by strengthening in the opposite direction when possible. But remember not to clench your teeth while exercising vigorously or lifting weights.

Variety is important when it comes to exercise, but be smart about changing gears. Make changes slowly and only progress as tolerated. You may need to modify some exercises or activities. For example, if you have neck pain, you may find it difficult to repeatedly turn your neck when doing the front-crawl swim stroke. If you enjoy aerobics but have a sore neck, you may need to avoid reaching overhead or modify the moves. If you love to snorkel, you might try sealing the mouthpiece with the lips to avoid clenching your jaw. Some sports may require you to use bite guards, but if they do, they are potentially hazardous to your jaw.

Summary

Stress is a natural part of life, but constant or too much stress is problematic and will aggravate jaw, neck, and head pain and dysfunction. Healthy movement and exercise also play an important role in healing. Your action plan should include both an exercise and stress-management program, and you must be sure to consider the following tips:

1. Learn to recognize and manage unhealthy stressors in your life.

2. It is important to slow down, mediate, seek balance, exercise, learn total body relaxation techniques, and breathe effortlessly through your nose and with your diaphragm.

3. Find and develop several stress management strategies that work for you and use them regularly.

4. Commit to an exercise program and work with your doctor or health-care provider to determine what is best for you and your health circumstances. Start slow and easy and increase as tolerated. Decide on a way to monitor the intensity, using either your pulse or a perceived exertion scale, and be sure to include a warm-up and cool-down period.

5. Decide what stretches and exercises are appropriate for you and stretch after you exercise.

6. Make yourself a checklist for change, based on the sample in Table 11.3 below.

Table 11.3: Checklist for Change: Stress Reduction and Exercise

HURTFUL HABIT	HEALTHY HABIT	CHECKLIST FOR CHANGE
I feel totally stressed and out-of-control most of the time, and I am always on the go.	I feel more in control. I make time to relax, meditate, and talk and laugh with family and friends. I have found stress management techniques that work for me and I use them.	I will simplify my life. I will learn to breathe, meditate, and make time for friends. I will find and develop stress management methods that help me switch gears when I am anxious, including breathing techniques.
I am a couch potato by night and a computer junkie by day. I get my exercise by walking to the refrigerator.	I make time to exercise regularly and have developed some hobbies that encourage me to move.	I will decide on an exercise program with my health-care provider. I will reward myself every week for the first month with a massage. I will sign up for a yoga class.
I walk every day, but I never stretch and have horrible posture.	I will stretch after walking. including using stretches that will improve my ability to maintain good postures.	I will design a stretching program with my physical therapist. I will think about adding variety to my exercise regime.

12

Step 10: Make Your Action Plan

Step 10 is the final step and involves creating an action plan. Have you heard the motto: "If you want to keep getting what you're getting, then keep doing what you're doing"? Well, your TMJ-related symptoms won't change unless you do. Now that you know the basics, it is time to implement whatever changes are needed for success. As my mother often said, "If you fail to plan, you plan to fail." Failing isn't an option, so it is time to make a plan.

What Do You Want to Change?

The best way to change a hurtful habit is to make a plan so you can replace it with a healthy one. Some of my patients have changed hurtful habits in as little as two weeks of consistent effort. However, keep in mind that you may have been swallowing incorrectly or slouching for years and it could take months to relearn and reprogram yourself to do it correctly without thinking about it. You must be diligent and review these principles weekly, then monthly, to prevent yourself from reverting back to your hurtful habits.

So let's discuss the elements of a general action plan and then you can modify it to fit your situation. I hope you made notes while you were reading, as suggested in Chapter 1, about the hurtful habits that are specific for you. You can use these notes as you make a plan to replace each hurtful habit with a healthy one and then implement your ideas with your favorite techniques. If you did not take notes, perhaps this review will jog your memory. The following seven elements were discussed in Steps 1 to 9. Review them now and decide which ones you need to include in your action plan.

1. PoTSB TLC

The only way to change habitual behaviors is to regularly make yourself aware of your unconscious habits. PoTSB TLC is a useful tool to help you become more aware of and to change your habits for the better. When you check your PoTSB TLC, you need to pause and check all seven of these important unconscious habits. If you need to make a correction, do it right then. Make sure your:

Po = **Po**sture is balanced
T = **T**ongue is anchored on "the spot"
S = **S**wallowing is correct
B = **B**reathing is relaxed through your nose and with your
diaphragm
TLC = **T**eeth are slightly apart, with **L**ips together, and **C**alm
muscles and mind

Be sure to include the ones you have problems with in your action plan. It may be too much to do all at once, so you should focus first on the hurtful habits that seem to most aggravate your symptoms. The following tips are some creative ways to remember to check your PoTSB TLC:

- Strategically place sticky notes saying "PoTSB TLC" wherever you will see them and be reminded to check your PoTSB TLC. Put them on your fridge, in your car, at work, by the bed, on the bathroom mirror, and on the TV or computer.

- Set your watch alarm to go off every hour to remind you to check your PoTSB TLC.

- Wear your watch or ring on the wrong finger and check your PoTSB TLC whenever you notice it.

- Polish one fingernail, and when you notice that one nail, check your PoTSB TLC.

- Remember to check your PoTSB TLC whenever you see a certain type or color of car.

- Any time you sit down, stand up, or walk through a doorway, check your PoTSB TLC.

- Any time you walk up or down the stairs, check your PoTSB TLC.

- Place a rock in your pocket and when you feel it, check your PoTSB TLC.

- Elicit help from a friend or partner to remind you regularly to check your PoTSB TLC.

Let's look at each of the seven PoTSB TLC areas and review some of the techniques you have learned. As you read through the list, choose the ones you wish to include in your action plan. If you haven't already done so, you may need to purchase a few items or set up your bed or work surfaces to practice some of these healthy habits. Write yourself a list or put a note on your computer or other area and don't remove it until you have made the necessary healthy changes.

Posture
The following are some techniques and exercises to help you change hurtful habits or postures:

- Ensure you have adequate back support wherever you sit most often.

- Set up your bed with an extra pillow to support your knees and for your arms during side sleeping.

- If you are a stomach sleeper, use a body pillow or stitch a ball into the front of your pajamas to keep you from rolling onto your stomach.

- Purchase headsets for your phones (home and cell) and use them, or use a speakerphone to avoid holding the phone to your ear with your shoulder.

- Ergonomically arrange your computer and work surfaces.

Tongue on "The Spot"

The following are some techniques and exercises to help you change hurtful tongue habits:

- Practice clucking.

- Practice saying "*T, D, N, L, S,* and *Z*" without your tongue pushing your front teeth, but going to the roof of your mouth instead.

- Do orbiting exercises in the mirror six times when you wash your hands.

Swallow Correctly

The following are some techniques and exercises to help you learn to swallow correctly:

- Do ten tongue push-ups every day using Corn Flakes or Cheerios until you can swallow properly.

- Try using a cup with a straw to practice swallowing water correctly throughout the day.

- Label a paper cup by the sink with "Swallow Right" and practice swallowing correctly when you brush your teeth.

Breathe Well

The following are some techniques and exercises to help you learn to breathe correctly:

- Practice breathing through your nose, using your diaphragm and not making your neck muscles get involved in doing the work.

- While lying down, breathe through your belly and sides relaxing your chest, and place your hand or a book on your stomach for feedback.

- Check your breathing regularly to make sure it is not shallow.

- If you tend to breathe too quickly, train yourself to breathe more slowly and effortlessly.

Teeth Apart, Lips Together, and Calm Your Muscles and Mind

The following are some techniques and exercises to help you change hurtful teeth and lip habits:

- Stop bracing, clenching, and grinding.
- Incorporate short upper lip stretches and exercises, if needed.
- Implement stress-reduction techniques.
- Use a splint, if needed.
- Calm your muscles by eliminating caffeine and incorporating proper breathing.

2. Trigger Points

Find and eliminate trigger points in your muscles. Determine what brought them on or what keeps them from getting better. Make necessary changes for long-term relief. Incorporate a stretching program to maintain your motion and keep trigger points from returning.

3. Stretching Routine

Develop and write out an exercise routine, including appropriate stretches and progressions, and schedule it as part of your week's routine.

4. Menu Plan

Plan a 1- to 2-week menu of jaw-friendly foods that you will enjoy.

5. Symptom Diary

Set up a symptom diary. Use this diary to track your triggers and rate your symptoms when they occur, and be sure to indicate any precipitating events. You can also track the effectiveness of treatments and find what works best for you.

6. Problem Solving

Problem solve when your symptoms increase so you can figure out how best to eliminate the cause. If it is too difficult to problem solve on your own, seek the advice of a qualified professional.

7. Review

Write a note on your calendar to review the principles from this book weekly, then monthly, until you know and fully understand each of the healthy habits and postures and which of your hurtful habits need to be replaced with healthy ones. Get help from a specialist if you are not making progress or if you need help in any areas.

Choosing a Provider and Seeing a Specialist

I have *introduced* each of the healthy habits, but you may not be able to *implement* them alone. You may need a variety of specialists to help you along the way. For example, most people we see at our clinic have been evaluated by a TMJ disorders expert who is a member of the American Board of Orofacial Pain to rule out infection or any serious underlying problems. Then they are evaluated by a physical therapist with years of experience in head, neck, and jaw disorders and given an individual physical therapy treatment plan. You may need a speech-language pathologist trained in tongue-thrust and swallowing disorders to help you with hurtful swallowing and tongue-thrust habits. You may have a serious jaw-joint problem or muscle imbalance that needs to be resolved by a dentist or a doctor who specializes in TMJ. Or you may need to see an ENT or allergist who can help open your airway, a sleep specialist if you have sleep apnea, or a counselor to help you overcome abuse issues. Whatever the case may be, it is still wise to set the stage for healing with these healthy habits. If you needed surgery or orthodontics, you would not want to revert to the hurtful habits that may have contributed to the problem in the first place or stop you from getting better quickly and completely. A recent *New England Journal of Medicine* report indicated that 85 to 90 percent of people with TMJ disorders could be treated with "noninvasive, nonsurgical and reversible interventions." Those who don't respond to a reasonable course of this type of nonsurgical intervention, generally within three to six months, may need to consider more serious options if the condition interferes with their normal activities and daily life. Some patients with serious joint problems, like a locked jaw, may need surgery early on.[1]

I cannot emphasize enough how important it is for you to do your homework before choosing a provider or undergoing treatment. It is best if you can see a professional who specializes in head, neck, and jaw dysfunction. The jaw joints are one of the most complex joints, and it is my opinion that head, neck, and jaw problems are probably the most difficult orthopedic condition to treat. I trained for two years and undertook intensive study and professional courses before independently working with this patient population.

It would be nice to believe that all health-care providers only care about your health and well-being. Most care very much, but there some who are sidetracked by secondary gain. Unfortunately, money and tunnel vision can get in the way. I have seen far too many patients undergo irreversible procedures and waste thousands of dollars and end up worse than when they started. You must explore the conservative and reversible options first and then always get a qualified independent second opinion before doing something irreversible or extremely expensive. My motto is "Measure twice, cut once." And the NIDCR says, "Less is often best."[2]

This book is an effort to educate you so that you can more easily navigate the system and make better choices. Unfortunately, insurance companies and professions have taken your body as a whole and divided it into parts, as if they function separately. Your mouth and teeth are generally assigned to dental professionals. Your head, neck, and other body parts are assigned to medical providers, and your psychological, social, and emotional health are assigned to mental health providers. However, none of these body parts works independently. Add to that the joints that closely and intricately involve all three areas of your body, and insurance companies and many health-care providers turn you away or mistreat you because it is not their "area." You must think of your body as a whole unit. But to treat all its parts, you may need to involve a team of professionals.

A Plea to Parents and Health-Care Professionals Working with Children and Young Adults

Hurtful habits developed and repeated as a child or as an adolescent can have permanent and often unfortunate and unnecessary ramifications. These habits can adversely affect how the bones and structures in the face and jaw develop, the arrangement of teeth, how breathing takes place, and how their posture develops. Although there is much that can be done as adults to reverse or minimize the impact of hurtful habits that developed during childhood, it is not always possible to completely undo damage done during these formative years.

My plea is for parents and any health-care professional treating children and young adults to be aware of these hurtful habits and to help parents, young people, and caregivers become aware of how critically important it is for them to establish healthy habits while they are young. I believe that teaching and encouraging these healthy habits will help stem the ever-growing tide of chronic TMJ-related problems. The potential for improving the child, or young person's, quality of life is huge. Parents must be aware that sucking on a thumb or pacifier in the formative years can alter the development of normal tongue position, swallowing, breathing, and even facial development. The healthy habits represented by the acronym PoTSB TLC should be taught by doctors, dentists, and hygienists at annual check-ups and by parents at bedtime.

Health-care practitioners should be on the lookout for people with hypermobile joints, educate them on joint protection measures, and send them to a physical therapist to get them on a program to stabilize and protect their joints. Parents and practitioners alike should take a more active role in encouraging healthy sleep, postures, and positions, and in encouraging an active lifestyle with lots of healthy movement.

Opening the airway is first principle in the ABCs of first aid. If children can't breathe through their noses, they are headed for problems. Enlarged tonsils, adenoids, narrow sinuses, upper-respiratory problems, and allergies must all be seriously considered and resolved as early as possible.

Jim: A Mouth Breather

A seventeen-year-old named Jim grew up breathing through his mouth because he had narrow sinuses. He suffered many upper respiratory and sinus infections during his formative years. His face, mouth, and jaw developed abnormally because of this, and now he is about to undergo several major surgeries that will, among other things, open his sinuses and realign his jaw in an effort to put things back in order.

Parents should also be aware of the long-term impact that early jaw joint injuries can have. Think twice before signing your child up for boxing, karate, football, or other contact sports. Always use appropriate protective gear, including mouth guards.

My hope is that this book will raise awareness so that intervention will be received while development is still occurring so that many of these situations can be prevented and avoided.

Conclusion

Thank you for joining me on this journey. In this book I have tried to empower you with as much information as possible about this condition so that you can take appropriate steps and make any necessary changes in your life to allow for healing to take place. Although there may not be a "cure" for the orthopedic problems in your jaw or neck, following the guidelines in this book should allow you to function with much less discomfort and dysfunction.

I hope and pray you will benefit from these principles and that you will spread the word. These healthy habits are good for the general population and not just for those with pain and dysfunction. Tell your family and friends about these healthy habits. Tell your doctor and dentist. Read this book at your book club and you can all practice swallowing, clucking, and doing tongue push-ups together.

Resources

American Academy of Sleep Disorders

www.sleepcenters.org

This website is provided by the American Academy of Sleep Disorders and will help you locate an *accredited sleep center* and laboratory members.

American Association of Oral and Maxillofacial Surgeons

www.aaoms.org/tmj.php

American Academy of Craniofascial Pain

www.aacfp.org

American Academy of Orofacial Pain

(856) 423-3629

www.aaop.org

This site offers several patient information handouts online and can help you locate a TMJ disorders expert in your area.

The American Chronic Pain Association

(800) 533-3231

www.theacpa.org

Provides information and support, including steps to managing chronic pain, links to groups, clinical trials and studies, and guidelines for choosing a chronic pain program.

American Dental Association

www.ada.org/public/topics/tmd_tmj.asp

American Physical Therapy Association

www.apta.org

Offers consumer brochures and information on how to find a physical therapist.

American Speech Language Hearing Association

(800) 638-8255

www.asha.org

If you need additional help in order to swallow correctly or eliminate a tongue thrust, this site can help you locate speech-language pathologists in your area to help you. However, you will need to ensure they specialize in the specific area(s) you need. Not all speech-language professionals are trained in tongue-thrust and swallowing disorders.

Cornell University Ergonomics Website
http://ergo.human.cornell.edu *and* http://healthycomputing.com
These websites provide instruction and ergonomic guidelines to help you set up all aspects of your workstation to minimize irritation to your body. It offers additional help for various ergonomic concerns like those who are left handed or use two screens.

The Jaw Joints and Allied Musculo-Skeletal Disorders Foundation
www.tmjoints.org
This is a nonprofit advocacy organization that promotes prevention, awareness, education, and research. The founders, Milton and Renee Glass, were successful in getting the month of November declared as National TMJ Awareness Month.

National Institute of Dental and Craniofacial Research: National Institutes of Health
www.nidcr.nih.gov/OralHealth/Topics/TMJ/TMJDisorders.htm

National Institutes of Health
www.nlm.nih.gov/medlineplus/ency/article/001227.htm

National Headache Foundation
(888) 643-5552
www.headaches.org
For a list of common foods that can trigger headaches refer to their Headache Diet: http://www.headaches.org/pdf/Diet.pdf.

National Fibromyalgia Association
www.fmaware.org

The TMJ Association
www.tmj.org
This association was founded by Terrie Cowley and Sandra Geilfuss. It is a nonprofit, patient-based advocacy group whose mission is to provide information on TMJ disorders to patients, health-care professionals, and the public and to advocate for research and treatment.

Notes

Introduction

1. Janet G. Travell and David G. Simons, *Myofascial Pain and Dysfunction: The Trigger Point Manual,* Vol. 1 (Baltimore, MD: Williams & Wilkins, 1983, 103).
2. Terrie Cowley, "Status of TMD Diagnosis and Treatment." Who We Are: TMJA Presentations/Letters. TMJ Association, http://www.tmj.org/061291.asp (accessed 14 April 2009). A public testimony presented 12 June 1991 to the National Institutes of Health Task Force on Opportunities for Research on Women's Health.
3. Steven J. Scrivani, David A. Keith, and Leonard B. Kaban, "Temporomandibular Disorders." *The New England Journal of Medicine* 359, no. 25 (2008): 2693–2705.
4. Michael E. Prater, Byron J. Bailey, and Francis B. Quinn, "Temporomandibular Joint Disorders," *Temporomandibular Joint Disorders* (March 1998), http://www.utmb.edu/otoref/grnds/tmj-1998/tmj.htm (accessed 14 April 2009); Richard B. Lipton and Marcelo E. Bigal, "Migraine and Other Headache Disorders," Scribd/Taylor & Francis Group, http://www.scribd.com/doc/8567521/Migraine-and-Other-Headache-Disorders (accessed 14 April 2009).
5. NIDCR National Institute of Health. "Less Is Often Best in Treating TMJ Disorders." http://www.nidcr.nih.gov/OralHealth/Topics/TMJ/LessisBest.htm (accessed 14 April 2009).
6. Scrivani, Keith, and Kaban, "Temporomandibular Disorders," 2693–2705.
7. National Institute of Dental and Craniofacial Research with NIH online pamphlet, "*TMJ Disorders,*" http://www.nidcr.nih.gov/OralHealth/Topics/TMJ/TMJDisorders.htm (accessed 14 April 2009).

Chapter 2
Important Anatomy

1. M. M. Panjabi and A. A. White III, *Biomechanics in the Musculoskeletal System* (New Haven, CT: Churchill Livingstone, 2001, 175)

2. Welden E. Bell, *Temporomandibular Disorders: Classification, Diagnosis, Management*, 3rd ed. (Chicago, IL: Year Book Medical Publishers, Inc., 1990).

3. Zarb et al. *Temporomandibular Joint and Masticatory Muscle Disorders*, 2nd ed. (Munksgaard, Copenhagen: Mosby, 1995)

4. H. Kang, G. J. Bao, and S. N. Qi, "Biomechanical Responses of Human Temporomandibular Joint Disc under Tension and Compression," *International Journal of Oral Maxillofacial Surgery* 35, no. 9 (September 2006): 817–21.

5. Jeffrey P. Okeson, *Managment of Temporomandibular Disorders and Occlusion*, 6th ed. (St. Louis, MO: Mosby Elsevier, 2008, 9).

6. Jeffrey P. Okeson, *Managment of Temporomandibular Disorders and Occlusion*, 6th ed. (St. Louis, MO: Mosby Elsevier, 2008).

7. J. Grönqvist, B. Häggman-Henrikson, and P. O. Eriksson, "Impaired Jaw Function and Eating Difficulties in Whiplash-associated Disorders," *Swedish Dentistry Journal*. 32, no. 4 (2008): 171–77; Bell, 1990.

8. Robert Berkow et al., eds., *The Merck Manual of Medical Information* (New York: Pocket Books, Simon & Schuster, 1997).

9. NINDS National Institute of Neurological Disorders and Stroke. "NINDS Occipital Neuralgia Information Page." http://www.ninds.nih.gov/disorders/occipitalneuralgia/occipitalneuralgia.htm (accessed 29 April 2009); Janet G. Travell and David G. Simons, *Myofascial Pain and Dysfunction: The Trigger Point Manual*, Vol. 1 (Baltimore, MD: Williams & Wilkins, 1983).

10. M. B. Yunus, "Central Sensitivity Syndromes: A New Paradigm and Group Nosology for Fibromyalgia and Overlapping Conditions, and the Related Issue of Disease Versus Illness," *Seminars in Arthritis and Rheumatism* 37 (June 2008): 339–52; P. Svensson, T. List, and G. Hector, "Analysis of Stimulus-evoked Pain in Patients with Myofascial Temporomandibular Pain Disorders," *Pain* 92, no. 3 (June 2001): 399–409.

11. Steven L. Kraus, *Temporomandibular Joint Disorders*, 2nd ed. (New York: Churchill Livingstone, Inc, 1994).

Chapter 3
Step 1: Stop the Overuse and Abuse of Your Jaw

1. Y. Zhao and D. Ye, "Measurement of Biting Force of Normal Teeth at Different Ages," *Hua Xi Yi Ke Da Xue Xue Bao* 25, no. 4 (1994): 414–17.

2. H. Kang, G. J. Bao, and S. N. Qi, "Biomechanical Responses of Hu-

man Temporomandibular Joint Disc under Tension and Compression," *International Journal of Oral and Maxillofacial Surgery* 35, no. 9 (September 2006): 817–21.

3. American Academy of Orofacial Pain. "Patient Information: TMD Tutorial." http://aaop.avenet.net/index.asp?type=B_BASIC&SEC= {5C4A7D2C-EFC8-450C-B93F-DCC0E8E640FD} (accessed 14 April 2009).

4. Rocabado, Mariano, and Z. Annette Iglarsh. *Musculoskeletal Approach to Maxillofacial Pain.* New York: J. B. Lippincott Company, 1991.

5. U.S. Dietary Health Guideline. http://www.health.gov/Dietary Guidelines (accessed 14 April 2009).

6. Travell, Janet G., and David G. Simons. *Myofascial Pain and Dysfunction: The Trigger Point Manual.* Vol. 1. Baltimore: Williams & Wilkins, 1983.

Chapter 4
Step 2: The Power of Posture: Learn How to Stand, Sit, and Sleep

1. Paul Brindza, "How Many Atoms Are in the Human Head?" Jefferson Lab, http://education.jlab.org/qa/mathatom_03.html (accessed 26 April 2009).

2. H. Duane Saunders, *Self-Help Manual For Your Neck* (Chaska, MN: The Saunders Group, Inc., 1992).

3. H. Ohmure et al., "Influence of Forward Head Posture on Condylar Position," *Journal of Oral Rehabilitation* 35, no. 11 (November 2008): 795–800.

4. Mariano Rocabado and Z. Annette Iglarsh, *Musculoskeletal Approach to Maxillofacial Pain* (New York: J.B. Lippincott Company, 1991).

5. Robert L. Talley, "TMD: An Orthopedic Perspective" (professional presentation, Dallas, TX, 26 January 2006).

6. Annette Iglarsh et al., "The Secret of Good Posture." (n.d.) http://www.apta.org/AM/Template.cfm?Section=Home&TEMPLATE=/CM/HTMLDisplay.cfm&CONTENTID=20457 (accessed 26 April 2009) and http://www.larsonrehab.com/downloads/Posture%20brochure%20apta.pdf (accessed 16 November 2009).

7. E. M. Tingey, P. H. Buschang, and G. S. Throckmorton, "Mandibular Rest Position: A Reliable Position Influenced by Head Support and Body Posture," *American Journal of Orthodontics and Dentofacial Orthopedics* 120, no. 6 (2001): 614–22.

8. O. Komiyama et al., "Posture Correction as Part of Behavioural Therapy in Treatment of Myofascial Pain with Limited Opening," *Journal of Oral Rehabilitation* 26, no. 5 (1999): 428–35.

9. P. H. Witherspoon, Jr., "Why Some Cases of Mandibular Advancement Fail," *Functional Orthodontist* 21, no. 2 (April–June 2004): 24–30, 32.

10. Mark A. Caselli and Edward C. Roznca, "Detecting and Treating Leg Length Discrepancies," *Podiatry Today* 15, no. 12 (2002), http://www.podiatrytoday.com/article/1035 (accessed 26 April 2009).

11. Janet G. Travell and David G. Simons, *Myofascial Pain and Dysfunction: The Trigger Point Manual*, Vol. 1 (Baltimore, MD: Williams & Wilkins, 1983).

12. David G. Magee, *Orthopedic Physical Assessment*, 4th ed. (St. Louis, MO: Saunders Elsevier, 2008).

13. Florence P. Kendall, *Muscles Testing and Function with Posture and Pain*, 5th ed. (Baltimore, MD: Lippincott Williams & Wilkins, 2005).

14. Magee, *Orthopedic Physical Assessment*.

15. D. A. Neumann, *Kinesiology of the Musculoskeletal System—Foundations for Physical Rehabilitation* (St. Louis, MO: C.V. Mosby, 2002).

16. H. Duane Saunders, *Evaluation, Treatment and Prevention of Musculoskeletal Disorders* (Minneapolis, MN: Viking Press, Inc., 1985, 317).

17. J. Lapointe et al., "Interaction Between Postural Risk Factors and Job Strain on Self-reported Musculoskeletal Symptoms among Users of Video Display Units: A Three-year Prospective Study," *Scandinavian Journal of Work and Environmental Health* 35, no. 2 (2009): 134–44.

18. Alan Hedge, "What Is the 'Best' Sitting Posture?" HealthyComputing.com, http://www.healthycomputing.com/articles/publish/news/What_is_the_Best_Sitting_Posture.shtml (accessed 26 April 2009).

19. Reid Connell et al., "Cervical Spine with Human Cadaver Dissection" (professional course, Oregon Health Sciences University, September 1990).

20. Alan Hedge, "Tips for Reducing Eye Strain," HealthyComputing.com, http://www.healthycomputing.com/articles/publish/tips/Tips_For_Reducing_Eyestrain.shtml (accessed 26 April 2009).

21. Graciela M. Perez, "Ten Tips to Improve Your Ergonomics While Driving," Los Alamos National Lab, http://www.lanl.gov/orgs/pa/newsbulletin/2004/05/17/ErgonomicsandDriving.pdf (accessed 26 April 2009).

22. Philip Fabrizio, "Ergonomic Intervention in the Treatment of a Pa-

tient with Upper Extremity and Neck Pain," *Physical Therapy* 89, no. 4 (April 2009): 351–60.

23. Alan Hedge, "Ergonomic Guidelines for Arranging a Computer Workstation—10 Steps for Users," http://ergo.human.cornell.edu/ergoguide.html (accessed 24 October 2009).

24. William C. Dement and Christopher Vaughn, *The Promise of Sleep* (New York: Delacorte Press, 1999).

25. Barry J. Sessle et al., eds., *Orofacial Pain*, 2nd ed. (Chicago, IL: Quintessence Publishing Co., 2008).

26. H. Yatani, "Comparison of Sleep Quality and Psychologic Characteristics in Patients with Temporomandibular Disorders," *Journal of Orofacial Pain* 16, no. 3 (2002): 221–28, http://www.ncbi.nlm.nih.gov/pubmed/12221738 (accessed 8 November 2009).

27. Sessle et al., *Orofacial Pain*, 130.

28. Travell and Simons, *Myofacial Pain*.

29. Richard Ferber, *Solve Your Child's Sleep Problems*, 2nd ed. (New York: Fireside, 2006).

30. *Consumer Reports on Health* 20, no. 11 (November 2008): 10.

31. "Your Guide to Healthy Sleep," NIH publication No. 06-5800, April 2006, http://www.nhlbi.nih.gov/health/public/sleep/healthysleepfs.pdf (accessed 26 April 2009).

32. National Institutes of Health, "Sleep Apnea," http://www.nlm.nih.gov/medlineplus/sleepapnea.html (accessed 27 April 2009).

33. Talley, "TMD."

Chapter 5
Step 3: TLC: Teeth Apart, Lips Together, and Calm Your Muscles and Mind

1. James L. Guinn, "TMD from A to Z" (professional course, Salt Lake City, UT, 1 November 2002).

2. Y. Zhao and D. Ye, "Measurement of Biting Force of Normal Teeth at Different Ages," *Hua Xi Yi Ke Da Xue Xue Bao* 25, no. 4 (1994): 414–17.

3. Guinn, "TMD A to Z."

4. Ibid.

5. Ibid.

6. Steven J. Scrivani, David A. Keith, and Leonard B. Kaban, "Temporomandibular Disorders," *The New England Journal of Medicine* 359, no. 25 (2008): 2693–2705.

7. Janet G. Travell and David G. Simons, *Myofascial Pain and Dysfunction: The Trigger Point Manual*, Vol. 1. (Baltimore, MD: Williams & Wilkins, 1983).

8. "A New Way for TMJ," *Harvard Health Letter*, February 2009. https://www.health.harvard.edu/newsletters/Harvard_Health_Letter/2009/February (accessed 1 February 2009).

9. Scrivani, Keith, and Kaban, "Temporomandibular Disorders."

10. M. Z. Al-Ani et al., "Stabilisation Splint Therapy for Temporomandibular Pain Dysfunction Syndrome," Cochrane Database of Systematic Reviews 2004, Issue 1, http://www.cochrane.org/reviews/en/ab002778.html (accessed 20 April 2009).

11. Scrivani, Keith, and Kaban, "Temporomandibular Disorders," 2701–02.

12. Mariano Rocabado and Z. Annette Iglarsh, *Musculoskeletal Approach to Maxillofacial Pain*. New York: J.B. Lippincott Company, 1991.

13. M. Rocabado, B. E. Johnston, and M. G. Blakney, "Physical Therapy and Dentistry: An Overview," *Journal of Craniomandibular Practice* 1, no. 1 (1982–1983): 47–49.

14. Rocabado and Iglarsh, *Musculoskeletal Approach*.

15. Harold Gelb, *Clinical Management of Head, Neck and TMJ Pain and Dysfunction: A Multi-Disciplinary Approach to Diagnosis and Treatment*, 2nd ed. (Philadelphia, PA: W.B. Saunders Company, 1985).

16. Ibid.

17. Theresa Hale, *Breathing Free* (New York: Harmony Books, 1999).

18. Gelb, *Clinical Management*.

Chapter 6
Step 4: Train Your Tongue and Swallow Carefully

1. C. Lazarus et al., "Effects of Two Types of Tongue Strengthening Exercises in Young Normals," *Folia Phoniatrica Et Logopaedica* 55, no. 4 (2003): 199–205.

2. Mariano Rocabado and Z. Annette Iglarsh, *Musculoskeletal Approach to Maxillofacial Pain* (New York: J. B. Lippincott Company, 1991).

3. E. P. Harvold, "The Role of Function in the Etiology and Treatment of Malocclusion," *American Journal of Orthodontics and Dentofacial Orthopedics* 54 (1968): 883–98; E. P. Harvold, K. Vargervik, and G. Chierici, "Primate Experiments on Oral Sensation and Dental

Malocclusions," *American Journal of Orthodontics and Dentofacial Orthopedics* 63 (1973): 494–508; E. P. Harvold et al., "Primate Experiments on Oral Respiration," *American Journal of Orthodontics and Dentofacial Orthopedics* 79, no. 4 (April 1981): 359–72; George P. Chierici, Egil Harvold, and W. James Dawson, "Primate Experiments on Facial Asymmetry," *Journal of Dental Research* 49 (July 1970): 847–51; K. Vargervik et al., "Morphologic Response to Changes in Neuromuscular Patterns Experimentally Induced by Altered Modes of Respiration," *American Journal of Orthodontics and Dentofacial Orthopedics* 85, no. 2 (February 1984): 115–24.

4. T. M. Weiss, S. Atanasov, and K. H. Calhoun, "The Association of Tongue Scalloping with Obstructive Sleep Apnea and Related Sleep Pathology," *Archives of Otolaryngology Head and Neck Surgery* 133 (2005): 966–71.

5. R. M. Mason, and W. R. Proffit, "The Tongue Thrust Controversy: Background and Recommendations," *Journal of Speech and Hearing Disorders* 39 (May 1974): 115–32.

6. K. Yamada et al., "A Case of Anterior Open Bite Developing during Adolescence," *Journal of Orthodontics* 28, no. 1 (March 2001): 19–24.

7. Hilary Wilson, speech-language pathologist (personal interview, 2008).

8. Ibid.

9. Rocabado and Iglarsh, *Musculoskeletal Approach.*

10. Reid Connell et al., "Cervical Spine with Human Cadaver Dissection" (professional course, Oregon Health Sciences University, September 1990).

11. A. H. Messner and M. L. Lalakea, "Ankyloglossia: Controversies in Management," *International Journal of Pediatric Otorhinolaryngology* 54 (31 August 2000): 123–31.

12. Wilson, personal interview.

13. Curtis S. Weiss, Mary E. Gordon, and Herold S. Lillywhite, *Clinical Management of Articulatory and Phonologic Disorders*, 2nd ed. (Baltimore, MD: Williams & Wilkins, 1987).

14. Wilson, personal interview; D. M. Ruscello et al., "Macroglossia: A Case Study," *Journal of Communication Disorders* 38, no. 2 (March–April 2005): 109–22.

15. Weiss, Gordon, and Lillywhite, *Clinical Management.*

16. Rocabado and Iglarsh, *Musculoskeletal Approach.*

17. Table adapted from Steven L. Kraus, *Temporomandibular Joint Disorders*, 2nd ed. (New York: Churchill Livingstone, Inc., 1994).
18. Kraus, *Temporomandibular Joint Disorders*.
19. N. J. Lass et al., *Handbook of Speech-Language Pathology and Audiology* (St. Louis, MO: B. C. Decker Inc., 1988).
20. Barry J. Sessle et al., eds., *Orofacial Pain*, 2nd ed. (Chicago, IL: Quintessence Publishing Co., 2008).
21. Rocabado and Iglarsh, *Musculoskeletal Approach*.
22. Wilson, personal interview.
23. Douglas H. Morgan et al., *Diseases of the Temporomandibular Apparatus, A Multidisciplinary Approach*, 2nd ed. (St. Louis, MO: C.V. Mosby, 1982).
24. Harold Gelb, *Clinical Management of Head, Neck and TMJ Pain and Dysfunction: A Multi-Disciplinary Approach to Diagnosis and Treatment*, 2nd ed. (Philadelphia: W.B. Saunders Company, 1985).
25. W. R. Proffit, B. B. Chastain, and L. A. Norton, "Linguopalatal Pressure in Children," *American Journal of Orthodontics and Dentofacial Orthopedics* 55 (1969): 154–66.

Chapter 7
Step 5: Breathe Well

1. C. Gilbert, "Clinical Applications of Breathing Regulation: Beyond Anxiety Management," *Behavior Modification* 27, no. 5 (Oct 2003): 692–709; Robert Fried, *Breathe Well, Be Well: A Program to Relieve Stress, Anxiety, Asthma, Hypertension, Migraine, and Other Disorders for Better Health* (Hoboken, NJ: John Wiley and Sons, Inc., 1999).
2. Robert Fried, *The Hyperventilation Syndrome, Research and Clinical Treatment* (Baltimore, MD: The John Hopkins University Press, 1987).
3. W. K. Amery, "Brain Hypoxia: The Turning-point in the Genesis of the Migraine Attack?" *Cephalalgia* 2, no. 2 (June 1982): 83–109.
4. NINDS of the NIH, "Headache: Hope Through Research," http://www.ninds.nih.gov/disorders/headache/detail_headache.htm (accessed 25 October 2009).
5. Gilbert, "Clinical Applications"; H. Folgering, "The Pathophysiology of Hyperventilation Syndrome," *Monaldi Archives of Chest Disease* 54, no. 4 (August 1999): 365–72.
6. R. A. Cluff, "Chronic Hyperventilation and Its Treatment by Physiotherapy: Discussion Paper," *Journal of the Royal Society of Medicine*, no. 77, (October 1984): 855–62.

7. Thomas R. Baechle and Roger W. Earle, eds., *Essentials of Strength Training and Conditioning*, National Strength and Conditioning Association, 2nd ed. (Champaign, IL: Human Kinetics, 2000).
8. Fried, *Breathe Well*, 26.
9. Cluff, "Chronic Hyperventilation."
10. NIH Medline Plus, "Obesity Hypoventilation Syndrome," http://www.nlm.nih.gov/medlineplus/ency/article/000085.htm (accessed 1 August 2009).
11. E. P. Harvold et al., "Primate Experiments on Oral Respiration," *American Journal of Orthodontics and Dentofacial Orthopedics* 79, no. 4 (April 1981): 359–72.
12. Janet G. Travell and David G. Simons, *Myofascial Pain and Dysfunction: The Trigger Point Manual*, Vol. 1 (Baltimore, MD: Williams & Wilkins, 1983).
13. Fried, *Breathe Well*.
14. Ibid.; Theresa Hale, *Breathing Free* (New York: Harmony Books, 1999).
15. R. Galiano, "The Ins and Outs of Breathing," *The Dallas Morning News* (21 September 2004): 3E.
16. E. A. Holloway and R. J. West, "Integrated Breathing and Relaxation Training (the Papworth Method) for Adults with Asthma in Primary Care: A Randomised Controlled Trial," *Thorax* 62, no. 12 (2007): 1039–1042.
17. Baechle and Earle, *Essentials of Strength*.
18. Cluff, "Chronic Hyperventilation."

Chapter 8
Step 6: Care for Your Muscles

1. D. J. Alvarez and P. G. Rockwell, "Trigger Points: Diagnosis and Management," *American Family Physician* 65, no. 4 (15 February 2002): 653–60; Douglas H. Morgan et al., *Diseases of the Temporomandibular Apparatus: A Multidisciplinary Approach*, 2nd ed. (St. Louis, MO: C.V. Mosby, 1982).
2. Figure adapted from H. Duane Saunders, *Self-Help Manual for Your Neck* (Chaska, MN: The Saunders Group, Inc., 1992).
3. W. P. Hanten et al., "Effectiveness of a Home Program of Ischemic Pressure Followed by Sustained Stretch for Treatment of Myofascial Trigger Points," *Physical Therapy* 80, no. 10 (October 2000): 997–1003.

4. Janet G. Travell and David G. Simons, *Myofascial Pain and Dysfunction: The Trigger Point Manual*, Vol. 1 (Baltimore, MD: Williams & Wilkins, 1983); David G. Simons, Janet G. Travell, and Lois S. Simons, *Travell & Simons' Myofascial Pain and Dysfunction: The Trigger Point Manual*, 2nd ed. (Baltimore, MD: Williams & Wilkins, 1999).

5. R. D. Gerwin, "A Review of Myofascial Pain and Fibromyalgia—Factors that Promote their Persistence," *Acupuncture in Medicine* 23, no. 3 (September 2005): 121–34.

6. Simons, Travell, and Simons, *Travell and Simons' Myofascial.*

7. Travell and Simons, *Myofascial Pain.*

8. Ibid.

9. Simons, Travell, and Simons, *Travell and Simons' Myofascial.*

10. Ibid.

11. J. M. McPartland, "Travell Trigger Points—Molecular and Osteopathic Perspectives," *Journal of the American Osteopathic Association* 104, No. 6 (June 2004): 244–49; Simons, Travell, and Simons, *Travell and Simons' Myofascial.*

12. Simons, Travell, and Simons, *Travell and Simons' Myofascial.*

13. McPartland, "Travell Trigger Points."

14. Travell and Simons, *Myofascial Pain.*

15. Travell and Simons, *Myofascial Pain.*

16. This table is partially modified and modeled after a list used in David G. Simons, Janet G. Travell, and Lois S. Simons, *Travell & Simons' Myofascial Pain and Dysfunction: The Trigger Point Manual*, 2nd ed. (Baltimore, MD: Williams & Wilkins, 1999).

17. Gerwin, "A Review of Myofascial Pain."

18. Hanten, "Effectiveness of a Home Program."

19. C. Fernández de las Peñas et al., "Myofascial Trigger Points and their Relationship to Headache: Clinical Parameters in Chronic Tension-type Headache," *Headache* 46, no. 8 (September 2006): 1264–72.

20. Saunders, *Self-Help Manual.*

21. Simons, Travell, and Simons, *Travell and Simons' Myofascial.*

22. Fernández de las Peñas et al., "Myofascial Trigger Points."

23. Saunders, *Self-Help Manual.*

24. Travell and Simons, *Myofascial Pain.*

25. Simons, Travell, and Simons, *Travell and Simons' Myofascial.*

26. Travell and Simons, *Myofascial Pain.*

27. Fernández de las Peñas et al., "Myofascial Trigger Points."

28. Travell and Simons, *Myofascial Pain.*

29. Simons, Travell, and Simons, *Travell and Simons' Myofascial.*

30. T. Ono et al., "Evaluation of Tongue-, Jaw-, and Swallowing-Related Muscle Coordination During Voluntarily Triggered Swallowing," *International Journal of Prosthodontics* 22, no. 4 (2009): 493–98.
31. Travell and Simons, *Myofascial Pain.*
32. Simons, Travell, and Simons, *Travell and Simons' Myofascial.*
33. Ibid.
34. K. Matsunaga et al., "An Anatomical Study of the Muscles that Attach to the Articular Disc of the Temporomandibular Joint," *Clinical Anatomy* 22, no. 8 (2009): 932–40.
35. Travell and Simons, *Myofascial Pain.*
36. Simons, Travell, and Simons, *Travell and Simons' Myofascial.*
37. Ono et al., "Evaluation of Tongue-."
38. Travell and Simons, *Myofascial Pain.*
39. Simons, Travell, and Simons, *Travell and Simons' Myofascial.*
40. Travell and Simons, *Myofascial Pain.*
41. Simons, Travell, and Simons, *Travell and Simons' Myofascial.*
42. Travell and Simons, *Myofascial Pain*; Simons, Travell, and Simons, *Travell and Simons' Myofascial.*
43. Travell and Simons, *Myofascial Pain.*
44. Ibid.
45. Simons, Travell, and Simons, *Travell and Simons' Myofascial.*
46. Fernández de las Peñas et al., "Myofascial Trigger Points."
47. Simons, Travell, and Simons, *Travell and Simons' Myofascial.*
48. Travell and Simons, *Myofascial Pain.*
49. Simons, Travell, and Simons, *Travell and Simons' Myofascial.*
50. American College of Rheumatology, "Fibromyalgia," http://www.rheumatology.org/public/factsheets/diseases_and_conditions/fibromyalgia.asp?aud=pat (accessed 9 April 2009).
51. D. Starlanyl and M. E. Copeland, *Fibromyalgia & Chronic Myofascial Pain Syndrome: A Survival Manual* (Oakland, CA: New Harbinger Publications, 1996).
52. American College of Rheumatology, "Criteria for the Classification of Fibromyalgia," 1990, http://www.nfra.net/Diagnost.htm (accessed 9 April 2009).
53. Steven L. Kraus, *Temporomandibular Joint Disorders*, 2nd ed. (New York: Churchill Livingstone, Inc., 1994).
54. National Institute of Arthritis and Musculoskeletal and Skin Diseases, "Fibromyalgia," http://www.niams.nih.gov/Health_Info/Fibromyalgia/default.asp (accessed 29 April 2009).
55. Gerwin, "A Review of Myofascial Pain."

Chapter 9
Step 7: Care for Your Disks and Ligamentous Structures

1. Jeffrey P. Okeson, *Managment of Temporomandibular Disorders and Occlusion*, 6th ed. (St. Louis, MO: Mosby Elsevier, 2008).

2. Mariano Rocabado and Z. Annette Iglarsh, *Musculoskeletal Approach to Maxillofacial Pain* (New York: J. B. Lippincott Company, 1991).

3. Tufts University, "TMJ4," http://iris3.med.tufts.edu/dentgross/lab guide/TMJ4.html (accessed 27 October 2009).

4. A. Isberg, S. E. Widmalm, and R. Ivarsson, "Clinical, Radiographic and Electromyographic Study of Patients with Internal Derangement of the Temporomandibular Joint," *American Journal of Orthodontics and Dentofacial Orthopedics* 88, no. 6 (1985): 453–60.

5. NIDCR of the NIH, "TMJ Disorders," http://www.nidcr.nih.gov/OralHealth/Topics/TMJ/TMJDisorders.htm (accessed 29 April 2009).

6. S. J. Scrivani, D. A. Keith, and L. B. Kaban, "Temporomandibular Disorders," *New England Journal of Medicine* 359 (2008): 2693–2705.

7. Rocabado and Iglarsh, *Musculoskeletal Approach*, 81.

8. Rocabado and Iglarsh, *Musculoskeletal Approach*.

9. Steven L. Kraus, *Temporomandibular Joint Disorders*, 2nd ed. (New York: Churchill Livingstone, Inc., 1994).

10. Table adapted from a table in David G. Magee, *Orthopedic Physical Assessment*, 4th ed. (St. Louis, MO: Saunders Elsevier, 2008).

11. American Academy of Orofacial Pain, "Patient Information: TMD Tutorial," http://aaop.avenet.net/index.asp?type=B_BASIC &SEC={BACACF0A-25A6-49E6-A6DB-10CD34992C0F} (accessed 29 April 2009).

12. C. Hirsch, M. T. John, and A. Stang, "Association Between Generalized Joint Hypermobility and Signs and Diagnoses of Temporomandibular Disorders," *European Journal of Oral Sciences* 116, no. 6 (December 2008): 525–30.

13. Michael R. Simpson, "Benign Joint Hypermobility Syndrome: Evaluation, Diagnosis, and Management," *Journal of the American Osteopathic Association* 106, no. 9 (September 2006): 531–36.

14. F. Malfait et al., "The Genetic Basis of the Joint Hypermobility Syndromes." *Rheumatology* 45, no. 5 (May 2006): 502–07.

15. Arthritis Research Campaign, "Joint Hypermobility," http://www.arc.org.uk/arthinfo/patpubs/6019/6019.asp (accessed 29 April 2009).

16. The Hypermobility Syndrome Association, "The Brighton Score—The New Diagnostic Criteria for HMS," http://www.hyper mobility.org/diagnosis.php (accessed 24 July 2009).

17. Arthritis Research Campaign, "Joint Hypermobility."

Chapter 10
Step 8: Halt Head and Neck Pain

1. NINDS of the NIH, "Headache Hope Through Research," http://www.ninds.nih.gov/disorders/headache/headachehope.pdf (accessed 29 April 2009).

2. National Institutes of Health, Medline Plus, "Headache," http://www.nlm.nih.gov/medlineplus/ency/article/003024.htm (accessed 29 April 2009).

3. R. B. Lipton et al., "Classification of Primary Headaches," *Neurology* 10, no. 63 (August 2004): 427–35.

4. Y. D. Fragoso et al., "Crying As a Precipitating Factor for Migraine and Tension-type Headache, *Sao Paulo Medical Journal* 121, no. 1 (2 Jan 2003): 31–33.

5. National Headache Association, "Low Tyramine Headache Diet," http://www.headaches.org/pdf/Diet.pdf (accessed 24 July 2009).

6. National Institutes of Health, Medline Plus, "Headache."

7. D. B. Matchar et al., "The Headache Management Trial: A Randomized Study of Coordinated Care," *Headache* 48, no. 9 (October 2008): 1294–1310.

8. *Consumer Reports on Health*, "Dealing with a Pain in the Neck," August 2008, 7.

9. Ibid.

10. J. L. Riley et al., "Self-care Behaviors Associated with Myofascial Temporomandibular Disorder Pain," *Journal of Orofacial Pain* 21, no. 3 (2007): 194–202.

11. Mariano Rocabado and Z. Annette Iglarsh. *Musculoskeletal Approach to Maxillofacial Pain*. New York: J.B. Lippincott Company, 1991.

12. Janet G. Travell and David G. Simons, *Myofascial Pain and Dysfunction: The Trigger Point Manual*, Vol. 1 (Baltimore, MD: Williams & Wilkins, 1983).

13. Rocabado and Iglarsh, *Musculoskeletal Approach*.

14. Ibid.

15. Ibid.

Chapter 11
Step 9: Reduce Stress and Begin to Exercise

1. S. J. Scrivani, D. A. Keith, and L. B. Kaban, "Temporomandibular Disorders," *The New England Journal of Medicine* 359, no. 25 (2008): 2693–2705; M. B. Yunus, "Central Sensitivity Syndromes: A New Paradigm and Group Nosology for Fibromyalgia and Overlapping Conditions, and the Related Issue of Disease Versus Illness," *Seminars in Arthritis and Rheumatism* 37, no. 6 (June 2008): 339–52.

2. Scrivani, Keith, and Kaban, "Temporomandibular Disorders."

3. Erica Goode, "The Heavy Cost of Stress," *The New York Times*, 17 December 2002, http://www.nytimes.com/2002/12/17/science/the-heavy-cost-of-chronic-stress.html?pagewanted=1 (accessed 2 August 2009); W. B. Salt, II, and E. H. Season, *Fibromyalgia and the Mind/Body/Spirit Connection* (Columbus, OH: Parkview Publishing, 2000).

4. Jon Kabat-Zinn, *Full Catastrophe Living: Using the Wisdom of Your Body and Mind to Face Stress, Pain, and Illness* (New York: Dell Publishing, 1990, 80).

5. Stephanie Gold, "Mind Your Body: A Higher Road to Relaxation," *Psychology Today* (July/August 2007). http://www.psychologytoday.com/articles/index.php?term=pto-4380.html&fromMod=popular_anxiety (accessed 30 April 2009).

6. Caroline Myss, *Why People Don't Heal, and How They Can* (New York: Harmony Books, 1997).

7. U.S. Department of Health and Human Resources, "Physical Activity Guidelines for Americans," http://www.health.gov/PAGuidelines/committeereport.aspx. A summary is also available: http://www.health.gov/paguidelines/guidelines/summary.aspx (accessed 24 July 2009).

8. G. A. Brenes et al., "Treatment of Minor Depression in Older Adults: A Pilot Study Comparing Sertraline and Exercise," *Aging and Mental Health* 11, no. 1 (January 2007): 61–8; D. Haaland et al., "Is Regular Exercise a Friend or Foe of the Aging Immune System? A Systematic Review," *Clinical Journal of Sport Medicine* 18, no. 6 (November 2008): 539–48; A. C. King et al., "Effects of Moderate-intensity Exercise on Polysomnographic and Subjective Sleep Quality in Older Adults with Mild to Moderate Sleep Complaints," *The Journals of Gerontology Series A: Biological Sciences and Medical Sciences Advance* 63, no. 9 (September 2008): 997–1004; T. Liu-Ambrose and M. Donaldson, "Exercise and Cognition in Older Adults: Is There

a Role for Resistance-Training Programs?" *British Journal of Sports Medicine* 43, no.1 (January 2009): 25–7; T. Schwager, "Exercise and the Brain," *Advance for Physical Therapists and PT Assistants* (16 June 2008): 28–9.

9. H. Besson et al., "Relationship Between Subdomains of Total Physical Activity and Mortality," *Medicine and Science in Sports and Exercise* 40, no. 11 (8 November 2008): 1909–15

10. Thomas R. Baechle and Roger W. Earle, eds., *Essentials of Strength Training and Conditioning*, National Strength and Conditioning Association, 2nd ed. (Champaign, IL: Human Kinetics, 2000).

11. U.S. Department of Health and Human Resources, "Physical Activity Guidelines."

12. Janet G. Travell and David G. Simons, *Myofascial Pain and Dysfunction: The Trigger Point Manual*, Vol. 1 (Baltimore, MD: Williams & Wilkins, 1983).

13. Baechle and Earle, *Essentials of Strength*.

Chapter 12
Step 10: Make Your Action Plan

1. S. J. Scrivani, D. A. Keith, and L. B. Kaban, "Temporomandibular Disorders," *The New England Journal of Medicine* 359, no. 25 (2008): 2693–2705.

2. National Institute of Dental and Craniofascial Research, NIH, "Less Is Often Best in Treating TMJ Disorders," http://www.nidcr.nih.gov/OralHealth/Topics/TMJ/LessisBest.htm (accessed 14 April 2009).

References

Al-Ani, M. Z., S. J. Davies, R. J. M. Gray, P. Sloan, and A. M. Glenny. 2004. Stabilisation splint therapy for temporomandibular pain dysfunction syndrome. *Cochrane Database of Systematic Reviews 2004*, Issue 1. http://www.cochrane.org/reviews/en/ab002778.html (accessed 20 April 2009).

Alvarez, D. J., and P. G. Rockwell. 2002. Trigger points: diagnosis and management. *American Family Physician* 65, no. 4: 653–60.

American Academy of Orofacial Pain. Patient information: TMD tutorial. http://aaop.avenet.net/index.asp?Type=B_BASIC&SEC={5C4A7 D2C-EFC8-450C-B93F-DCC0E8E640FD} (accessed 14 April 2009).

American College of Rheumatology. 1990. Criteria for the classification of fibromyalgia. http://www.nfra.net/Diagnost.htm (accessed 9 April 2009).

American College of Rheumatology. Fibromyalgia. http://www.rheuma tology.org/public/factsheets/diseases_and_conditions/fibromyalgia .asp?aud=pat (accessed 9 April 2009).

Amery, W. K. 1982. Brain hypoxia: the turning-point in the genesis of the migraine attack? *Cephalalgia* 2, no. 2: 83–109.

A new way for TMJ. 2009. *Harvard Health Letter*. https://www.health .harvard.edu/newsletters/Harvard_Health_Letter/2009/February (accessed 1 February 2009).

Arthritis Research Campaign. Joint hypermobility. http://www.arc.org .uk/arthinfo/patpubs/6019/6019.asp (accessed 29 April 2009).

Astrand, P. O. 1987. Exercise physiology and its role in disease prevention and in rehabilitation. *Archives of Physical Medicine and Rehabilitation* 68:305–09.

Avitzur, Orly. 2008. Tracking down migraine triggers. *Consumer Reports on Health* 20, no. 4: 11.

Bacci, I., and M. Richman. 2002. Waiting to inhale. *Advance for Physical Therapists & PT Assistants*:32–34.

Baechle, Thomas R., and Roger W. Earle, eds. 2000. *Essentials of strength training and conditioning*. National Strength and Conditioning Association. 2nd ed. Champaign, IL: Human Kinetics.

Bell, Welden E. 1990. *Temporomandibular disorders: classification, diagnosis, management*. 3rd ed. Chicago, IL: Year Book Medical Publishers, Inc.

Berkow, Robert, Mark H. Beers, and Andrew J. Fletcher, eds. 1997. *The Merck manual of medical information*. New York: Pocket Books.

Besson, H., U. Ekelund, S. Brage, R. Luben, S. Bingham, K. T. Khaw, and N. J. Wareham. 2008. Relationship between subdomains of total physical activity and mortality. *Medicine and Science in Sports and Exercise* 40, no.11: 1909–15

Brazeau, G. A., H. A. Gremillion, C. G. Widmer, P. E. Mahan, M. B. Benson, A. P. Mauderli, J. L. Riley III, and C. L. Smith. 1998. The role of pharmacy in the management of patients with temporomandibular disorders and orofacial pain. *Journal of the American Pharmacy Association* 38:354–63.

Brenes, G. A., J. D. Williamson, S. P. Messier, W. J. Rejeski, M. Pahor, E. Ip, and B. W. Penninx. 2007. Treatment of minor depression in older adults: a pilot study comparing Sertraline and exercise. *Aging and Mental Health* 11, no. 1: 61–8.

Brindza, Paul. How many atoms are in the human head? Jefferson Lab. http://education.jlab.org/qa/mathatom_03.html (accessed 26 April 2009).

Bruce, B., J. F. Fries, and D. P. Lubeck. 2005. Aerobic exercise and its impact on musculoskeletal pain in older adults: A 14-year prospective, longitudinal. *Arthritis Research and Therapy* 7, no. 6: 1263–70.

Caselli, Mark A., and Edward C. Roznca. 2002. Detecting and treating leg length discrepancies. *Podiatry Today* 15, no. 12. http://www.podiatry today.com/article/1035 (accessed 26 April 2009).

Center on Aging Studies. Breathing exercises. University of Missouri-Kansas City. http://cas.umkc.edu/casww/brethexr.htm (accessed 27 April 2009).

Chierici, George P. Egil Harvold, and W. James Dawson. 1970. Primate experiments on facial asymmetry. *Journal of Dental Research* 49: 847–51.

Cluff, R. A. 1984. Chronic hyperventilation and its treatment by physiotherapy: discussion paper. *Journal of the Royal Society of Medicine,* no. 77: 855–62.

Connell, Reid, Jeffrey Flemming, John Oldham, and Ann Porter Hoke. 1990. Cervical spine with human cadaver dissection. Professional course, Oregon Health Sciences University.

Consumer Reports on Health. 2008. Vol. 20, no. 11: 10.

Consumer Reports on Health. 2008. Dealing with a pain in the neck. 7.

Cooper, S. 2003. Effect of two breathing exercises (Buteyko and pranayama) in asthma: a randomised controlled trial. *Thorax* 58, no. 8: 674–79.

Cowley, Terrie. Status of TMD diagnosis and treatment. Who we are: TMJA presentations/letters. TMJ Association. http://www.tmj.org/061291.asp (accessed 14 April 2009). A public testimony presented 12 June 1991 to the National Institutes of Health Task Force on Opportunities for Research on Women's Health.

Davis County Schools Communication Interventions. *Sound production ideas.* http://www.davis.k12.ut.us/studentserv/LCMT/SiSS%20Hyper link%20Documents/communication%20Interventions/sound%20 production%20ideas.pdf (accessed 28 April 2009).

Dement, William C., and Christopher Vaughn. 1999. *The promise of sleep.* New York: Delacorte Press.

Dimitroulis, G. 2005. The prevalence of osteoarthrosis in cases of advanced internal derangement of the temporomandibular joint: a clinical, surgical and histological study. *International Journal of Oral Maxillofacial Surgery* 34, no. 4: 345–49.

Fabrizio, Philip. 2009. Ergonomic intervention in the treatment of a patient with upper extremity and neck pain. *Physical Therapy* 89, no. 4: 351–60.

Ferber, Richard. 2006. *Solve your child's sleep problems.* 2nd ed. New York: Fireside.

Fernández de las Peñas, C., C. Alonso-Blanco, M. L. Cuadrado, R. D.

Gerwin, and J. A. Pareja. 2006. Myofascial trigger points and their relationship to headache: clinical parameters in chronic tension-type headache. *Headache* 46, no. 8: 1264–72.

———. 2006. Trigger points in the suboccipital muscles and forward head posture in tension-type headache. *Headache* 46, no. 3: 454–60.

Folgering, H. 1999. The pathophysiology of hyperventilation syndrome. *Monaldi Archives of Chest Disease* 54, no. 4: 365–72.

Fragoso, Y. D., L. Carvalho, F. Ferrero, D. M. Lourenço, and E. R. Paulino. 2003. Crying as a precipitating factor for migraine and tension-type headache. *Sao Paulo Medical Journal* 121, no 1: 31–33.

Fried, Robert. 1999. *Breathe well, be well: a program to relieve stress, anxiety, asthma, hypertension, migraine, and other disorders for better health.* Hoboken, NJ: John Wiley and Sons, Inc.

Fried, Robert. 1987. *The hyperventilation syndrome, research and clinical treatment.* Baltimore, MD: The John Hopkins University Press.

Fumal, A., and J. Schoenen. 2008. Tension-type headache: current research and clinical management. *The Lancet Neurology* 7, no. 1: 70–83.

Galiano, R. 2004. The ins and outs of breathing. *The Dallas Morning News* (21 September 2004): 3E.

Gelb, Harold. 1985. *Clinical management of head, neck and TMJ pain and dysfunction: a multi-disciplinary approach to diagnosis and treatment.* 2nd ed. Philadelphia, PA: W.B. Saunders Company.

Gerwin, R. D. 2005. A review of myofascial pain and fibromyalgia—factors that promote their persistence. *Acupuncture in Medicine* 23, no. 3: 121–34.

Gilbert. C. 2003. Clinical applications of breathing regulation: beyond anxiety management. *Behavior Modification* 27, no. 5: 692–709.

Gold, Stephanie. 2007. Mind your body: a higher road to relaxation. *Psychology Today.* http://www.psychologytoday.com/articles/index.php?term=pto-4380.html&fromMod=popular_anxiety (accessed 30 April 2009).

Goode, Erica. 2002. The heavy cost of stress. *The New York Times.* 17 December 2002. http://www.nytimes.com/2002/12/17/science/the-heavy-cost-of-chronic-stress.html?pagewanted=1 (accessed 2 August 2009).

Grönqvist, J. B. Häggman-Henrikson, and P. O. Eriksson. 2008. Impaired jaw function and eating difficulties in whiplash-associated disorders. *Swedish Dentistry Journal* 32, no. 4: 171–77.

Guinn, James L. 2002. *TMD from A to Z.* Professional course. Salt Lake City, UT.

Haaland, D. A., T. F. Sabljic, D. A. Baribeau, I. M. Mukovozov, and L. E. Hart. 2008. Is regular exercise a friend or foe of the aging immune system? A systematic review. *Clinical Journal of Sport Medicine* 18, no. 6: 539–48.

Hale, Theresa. 1999. *Breathing free.* New York: Harmony Books.

Hanten, W. P., S. L. Olson, N. L. Butts, and A. L. Nowicki. 2000. Effectiveness of a home program of ischemic pressure followed by sustained stretch for treatment of myofascial trigger points. *Physical Therapy* 80, no. 10: 997–1003.

Harvold, E. P. 1968. The role of function in the etiology and treatment of malocclusion. *American Journal of Orthodontics and Dentofacial Orthopedics* 54:883–98.

Harvold, E. P., K. Vargervik, and G. Chierici. 1973. Primate experiments on oral sensation and dental malocclusions. *American Journal of Orthodontics and Dentofacial Orthopedics* 63:494–508.

Harvold, E. P., B. S. Tomer, K. Vargervik, and G. Chierici. 1981. Primate experiments on oral respiration. *American Journal of Orthodontics and Dentofacial Orthopedics* 79, no. 4: 359–72.

Hedge, Alan. Tips for reducing eye strain. HealthyComputing.com. http://www.healthycomputing.com/articles/publish/tips/Tips_For _Reducing_Eyestrain.shtml (accessed 26 April 2009).

Hedge, Alan. Ergonomic guidelines for arranging a computer workstation—10 steps for users. http://ergo.human.cornell.edu/ergoguide .html (accessed 24 October 2009).

Hedge, Alan. What is the "best" sitting posture? HealthyComputing. com., http://www.healthycomputing.com/articles/publish/news/ What_is_the_Best_Sitting_Posture.shtml (accessed 26 April 2009).

Hirsch, C., M. T. John, and A. Stang. 2008. Association between generalized joint hypermobility and signs and diagnoses of temporomandibular disorders. *European Journal of Oral Sciences* 116, no. 6: 525–30.

Holloway, E. A., and R. J. West. 2007. Integrated breathing and relaxation training (the Papworth method) for adults with asthma in primary care: a randomised controlled trial. *Thorax* 62, no. 12: 1039–1042.

Huang, F., L. Miao, Y. J. Chen, and J. Chen. 2008. Study of the influence of emotional stress on mechanical hyperalgesia of masseter muscles in rats. *Hua Xi Kou Qiang Yi Xue Za Zhi* 26, no. 3: 320–23.

Hutcherson, C. A., E. M. Seppala, and J. J. Gross. 2008. Loving-kindness meditation increases social connectedness. *Emotion* 8, no. 5: 720–24.

The Hypermobility Syndrome Association. The Brighton score—the new diagnostic criteria for HMS. http://www.hypermobility.org/diagnosis .php (accessed 24 July 2009).

Iglarsh, Annette, Florence Kendall, Carole Lewis, and Shirley Sahrmann. n.d. The secret of good posture. http://www.apta.org/AM/Template. cfm?Section=Home&TEMPLATE=/CM/HTMLDisplay.cfm&CON TENTID=20457 (accessed 26 April 2009) and http://www.larsonre hab.com/downloads/Posture%20brochure%20apta.pdf (accessed 16 November 2009).

Isberg, A., S. E. Widmalm, and R. Ivarsson. 1985. Clinical, radiographic and electromyographic study of patients with internal derangement of the temporomandibular joint. *American Journal of Orthopedics* 88, no. 6: 453–60.

Kabat-Zinn, Jon. 1990. *Full catastrophe living: using the wisdom of your body and mind to face stress, pain, and illness.* New York: Dell Publishing, 80.

Kang, H., G. J. Bao, and S. N. Qi. 2006. Biomechanical responses of human temporomandibular joint disc under tension and compression. *International Journal of Oral Maxillofacial Surgery* 35, no. 9: 817–21.

Kendall, Florence P. 2005. *Muscles Testing and Function with Posture and Pain.* 5th ed. Baltimore, MD: Lippincott Williams & Wilkins.

King, A. C., K. Baumann, P. O'Sullivan, S. Wilcox, and C. Castro. 2008. Effects of moderate-intensity exercise on polysomnographic and subjective sleep quality in older adults with mild to moderate sleep complaints. *The Journals of Gerontology Series A: Biological Sciences and Medical Sciences Advance* 63, no. 9: 997–1004.

Kokkonen, J., A. G. Nelson, C. Eldredge, and J. B. Winchester. 2007. Chronic static stretching improves exercise performance. *Medicine and Science in Sports and Exercise* 39, no. 10: 1825–31.

Komiyama, O., M. Kawara, M. Arai, T. Asano, and K. Kobayashi. 1999. Posture correction as part of behavioural therapy in treatment of myofascial pain with limited opening. *Journal of Oral Rehabilitation* 26, no. 5: 428–35.

Kraus, Steven L. 1994. *Temporomandibular joint disorders.* 2nd ed. New York: Churchill Livingstone, Inc.

Lapointe, J., C. E. Dionne, C. Brisson, and S. Montreuil. 2009. Interaction between postural risk factors and job strain on self-reported musculoskeletal symptoms among users of video display units: a three-year prospective study. *Scandinavian Journal of Work and Environmental Health* 35, no. 2: 134–44.

Lass, N. J., L. V. McReynolds, J. L. Northern, and D. E. Yoder. 1988. *Handbook of speech-language pathology and audiology.* St. Louis, MO: B. C. Decker Inc.

Lazarus, C., J. A. Logemann, C. Huang, and A. W. Rademaker. 2003. Effects of two types of tongue strengthening exercises in young normals. *Folia Phoniatrica Et Logopaedica* 55, no. 4: 199–205.

Lipton, Richard B., and Marcelo E. Bigal, eds. 2006. Migraine and other headache disorders. Scribd/Taylor & Francis Group. http://www.scribd.com/doc/8567521/Migraine-and-Other-Headache-Disorders (accessed 14 April 2009).

Lipton, R. B., M. E. Bigal, T. J. Steiner, S. D. Silberstein, and J. Olesen. 2004. Classification of primary headaches. *Neurology* 10, no. 63: 427–35.

Liu-Ambrose, T., and M. Donaldson. 2009. Exercise and cognition in older adults: Is there a role for resistance-training programs? *British Journal of Sports Medicine* 43, no. 1: 25–7.

Magee, David G. 2008. *Orthopedic physical assessment.* 4th ed. St. Louis, MO: Saunders Elsevier.

Malfait, F., A. J. Hakim, A. De Paepe, and R. Grahame. 2006. The genetic basis of the joint hypermobility syndromes. *Rheumatology* 45, no. 5: 502–07.

Mason, R. 1979. Tongue thrust oral motor behavior: impact on oral conditions and dental treatment. Proceedings of the Workshop. U.S. Department of Health, Education, and Welfare, Public Health Service, National Institutes of Health.

Mason, R. M., and W. R. Proffit. 1974. The tongue thrust controversy: background and recommendations. *Journal of Speech and Hearing Disorders* 39:115–32.

Matchar, D. B., L. Harpole, G. P. Samsa, A. Jurgelski, R. B. Lipton, S. D. Silberstein, W. Young, S. Kori, and A. Blumenfeld. 2008. The headache management trial: a randomized study of coordinated care. *Headache* 48, no. 9: 1294–1310.

Matsunaga, K., A. Usui, K. Yamaguchi, and K. Akita. 2009. An anatomical study of the muscles that attach to the articular disc of the temporomandibular joint. *Clinical Anatomy* 22, no. 8 : 932–40.

McPartland, J. M. 2004. Travell trigger points—molecular and osteopathic perspectives. *Journal of the American Osteopathic Association* 104, no. 6: 244–49.

Messner, A. H., and M. L. Lalakea. 2000. Ankyloglossia: controversies in management. *International Journal of Pediatric Otorhinolaryngology* 54:123–31.

Mohl, N. 1977. Head posture and its role in occlusion. *International Journal of Orthodontics* 15, no. 1: 6–14.

Morgan, Douglas H., Leland R. House, William P. Hall, and S. James Vamas. 1982. *Diseases of the temporomandibular apparatus, a multidisciplinary approach.* 2nd ed. St. Louis, MO: C.V. Mosby.

Myss, Caroline. 1997. *Why people don't heal, and how they can.* New York: Harmony Books.

National Headache Association. Low tyramine headache diet. http://www.headaches.org/pdf/Diet.pdf (accessed 24 July 2009).

National Institute of Arthritis and Musculoskeletal and Skin Diseases. Fibromyalgia. http://www.niams.nih.gov/Health_Info/Fibromyalgia/default.asp (accessed 29 April 2009).

National Institute of Dental and Craniofacial Research with NIH online pamphlet. *TMJ disorders.* http://www.nidcr.nih.gov/OralHealth/Topics/TMJ/TMJDisorders.htm (accessed 14 April 2009).

National Institutes of Health. 2006. Your guide to healthy sleep. NIH publication no. 06-5800. http://www.nhlbi.nih.gov/health/public/sleep/healthysleepfs.pdf (accessed 26 April 2009).

National Institutes of Health. Headache. http://www.nlm.nih.gov/med lineplus/ency/article/003024.htm (accessed 29 April 2009).

National Institutes of Health. Sleep apnea. http://www.nlm.nih.gov/med lineplus/sleepapnea.html (accessed 27 April 2009).

Neumann, D. A. 2002. *Kinesiology of the musculoskeletal system—foundations for physical rehabilitation.* St. Louis, MO: C.V. Mosby.

NIDCR National Institutes of Health. TMJ disorders. http://www.nidcr.nih.gov/OralHealth/Topics/TMJ/TMJDisorders.htm (accessed 29 April 2009).

NIDCR National Institutes of Health. 2009. Less is often best in treating TMJ disorders. http://www.nidcr.nih.gov/OralHealth/Topics/TMJ/LessisBest.htm (accessed 14 April 2009).

NIH Medline Plus. Obesity hypoventilation syndrome. http://www.nlm.nih.gov/medlineplus/ency/article/000085.htm (accessed 1 August 2009).

NINDS National Institute of Neurological Disorders and Stroke. NINDS occipital neuralgia information page. http://www.ninds.nih.gov/disorders/occipitalneuralgia/occipitalneuralgia.htm (accessed 29 April 2009).

NINDS of the NIH. Headache: hope through research. http://www.ninds.nih.gov/disorders/headache/detail_headache.htm (accessed 25 October 2009).

Ohmure, H., S. Miyawaki, J. Nagata, K. Ikeda, K. Yamasaki, and A. Al-Kalaly. 2008. Influence of forward head posture on condylar position. *Journal of Oral Rehabilitation* 35, no. 11: 795–800.

Okeson, Jeffrey P. 2008. *Managment of temporomandibular disorders and occlusion.* 6th ed. St. Louis, MO: Mosby Elsevier.

Ono, T., H. Iwata, K. Hori, K. Tamine, J. Kondoh, S. Hamanaka, and M. Yoshinobu. 2009. Evaluation of tongue-, jaw-, and swallowing-related muscle coordination during voluntarily triggered swallowing. *International Journal of Prosthodontics* 22, no. 4: 493–98.

Panjabi, M. M., and A. A. White III. 2001. *Biomechanics in the musculo-skeletal system*. New Haven, CT: Churchill Livingstone, 175.

Perez, Graciela M. Ten tips to improve your ergonomics while driving. Los Alamos National Lab. http://www.lanl.gov/orgs/pa/newsbulletin/2004/05/17/ErgonomicsandDriving.pdf (accessed 26 April 2009).

Prater, Michael E., Byron J. Bailey, and Francis B. Quinn. 1998. Temporomandibular joint disorders. *Temporomandibular Joint Disorders*. http://www.utmb.edu/otoref/grnds/tmj-1998/tmj.htm (accessed 14 April 2009)

Proffit, W. R., B. B. Chastain, and L. A. Norton. 1969. Linguopalatal pressure in children. *American Journal of Orthodontics and Dentofacial Orthopedics* 55: 154–66.

Riley, J. L., C. D. Myers, T. P. Currie, O. Mayoral, R. G. Harris, J. A. Fisher, H.A. Gremillion, and M. E. Robinson. 2007. Self-care behaviors associated with myofascial temporomandibular disorder pain. *Journal of Orofacial Pain* 21, no. 3: 194–202.

Roach, Peter. 2004. *English phonetics and phonology*. New York: Cambridge University Press.

Rocabado, M., B. E. Johnston, and M. G. Blakney. 1982–1983. Physical therapy and dentistry: an overview. *Journal of Craniomandibular Practice* 1, no. 1: 47–49.

Rocabado, Mariano, and Z. Annette Iglarsh. 1991. *Musculoskeletal approach to maxillofacial pain*. New York: J. B. Lippincott Company.

Rocabado, Mariano. 1983. Arthrokinematics of the temporomandibular joint. *Dental Clinics of North America* 27, no. 3: 573–594.

Ruscello, D. M., C. Douglas, T. Tyson, and M. Durkee. 2005. Macroglossia: a case study. *Journal of Communication Disorders* 38, no. 2: 109–22.

Salt, W. B. II, and E. H. Season. 2000. *Fibromyalgia and the mind/body/spirit connection*. Columbus, OH: Parkview Publishing.

Saunders, H. Duane. 1985. *Evaluation, treatment and prevention of musculoskeletal disorders*. Minneapolis, MN: Viking Press, Inc., 317.

Saunders, H. Duane. 1992. *Self-help manual for your neck*. Chaska, MN: The Saunders Group, Inc.

Schwager, T. 2008. Exercise and the brain. *Advance for Physical Therapists and PT Assistants*: 28–9.

Scrivani, Steven J., David A. Keith, and Leonard B. Kaban. 2008. Temporomandibular disorders. *The New England Journal of Medicine* 359, no. 25: 2693–2705.

Senior, R. 2008. Follow these rules. *ADVANCE for Physical Therapists and PT Assistants* 19, no. 24: 20–21.

Sessle, Barry J., Gilles J. Lavigne, James P. Lund, and Ronald Dubner, eds. 2008. *Orofacial pain*. 2nd ed. Chicago, IL: Quintessence Publishing Co.

Simons, David G., Janet G. Travell, and Lois S. Simons. 1999. *Travell & Simons' myofascial pain and dysfunction: the trigger point manual*. 2nd ed. Baltimore, MD: Williams & Wilkins.

Simpson, Michael R. 2006. Benign joint hypermobility syndrome: evaluation, diagnosis, and management. *Journal of the American Osteopathic Association* 106, no. 9: 531–36.

Starlanyl, D., and M. E. Copeland. 1996. *Fibromyalgia & chronic myofascial pain syndrome: a survival manual*. Oakland, CA: New Harbinger Publications.

Svensson, P., T. List, and G. Hector. 2001. Analysis of stimulus-evoked pain in patients with myofascial temporomandibular pain disorders. *Pain* 92, no. 3: 399–409.

Talley, Robert L. 2006. TMD: an orthopedic perspective. Professional presentation, Dallas, TX.

Tingey, E. M., P. H. Buschang, and G. S. Throckmorton. 2001. Mandibular rest position: a reliable position influenced by head support and body posture. *American Journal of Orthodontics and Dentofacial Orthopedics* 120, no. 6: 614–22.

Travell, Janet G., and David G. Simons. 1983. M*yofascial pain and dysfunction: the trigger point manual*. Vol. 1. Baltimore, MD: Williams & Wilkins.

Tufts University. TMJ4. http://iris3.med.tufts.edu/dentgross/labguide/TMJ4.html (accessed 27 October 2009).

U.S. Department of Health and Human Resources. Physical activity guidelines for Americans. http://www.health.gov/PAGuidelines/committeereport.aspx. A summary is also available: http://www.health.gov/paguidelines/guidelines/summary.aspx (accessed 24 July 2009).

U.S. Dietary Health Guidelines. http://www.health.gov/DietaryGuide lines (accessed 14 April 2009).

Vargervik, K. A., J. Miller, G. Chierici, E. Harvold, and B. S. Tomer. 1984. Morphologic response to changes in neuromuscular patterns experimentally induced by altered modes of respiration. *American Journal of Orthodontics and Dentofacial Orthopedics* 85, no. 2: 115–24.

Weiss, Curtis S., Mary E. Gordon, and Herold S. Lillywhite. 1987. *Clinical management of articulatory and phonologic disorders.* 2nd ed. Baltimore, MD: Williams & Wilkins.

Weiss T. M., S. Atanasov, and K. H. Calhoun. 2005. The association of tongue scalloping with obstructive sleep apnea and related sleep pathology. *Archives of Otolaryngology Head and Neck Surgery* 133: 966–71.

Wilson, Hilary. 2008. Speech-language pathologist. Personal interview.

Witherspoon, P. H., Jr. 2004. Why some cases of mandibular advancement fail. *Functional Orthodontist* 21, no. 2: 24–30, 32.

Yamada, K., Y. Satou, K. Hanada, T. Hayashi, and J. Ito. 2001. A case of anterior open bite developing during adolescence. *Journal of Orthodontics* 28, no. 1: 19–24.

Yatani, H. 2002. Comparison of sleep quality and psychologic characteristics in patients with temporomandibular disorders. *Journal of Orofacial Pain* 16, no. 3: 221–28. http://www.ncbi.nlm.nih.gov/pubmed/ 12221738 (accessed 8 November 2009).

Yunus, M. B. 2008. Central sensitivity syndromes: a new paradigm and group nosology for fibromyalgia and overlapping conditions, and the related issue of disease versus illness. *Seminars in Arthritis and Rheumatism* 37:339–52.

Zhao, Y., and D. Ye. 1994. Measurement of biting force of normal teeth at different ages. *Hua Xi Yi Ke Da Xue Xue Bao* 25, no. 4: 414–17.

Zarb, George A., Gunnar E. Carlsson, Barry J. Sessle, and Norman D. Mohl. 1995. *Temporomandibular joint and masticatory muscle disorders.* 2nd ed. Munksqaard, Copenhagen: Mosby

Index

A

alcohol, 62, 64, 186–187, 203

allergies, 76, 89, 100, 118, 126, 225–227; to food, 112, 118, 184, 187, 190; testing, 184. *See also* diet, allergies

alveolar, 86, 86–88, 92–93, 97, 101, 104; consonants, 92; ridges, 86, 93, 96–97

American Board of Orofacial Pain (ABOP), *xi*, 275

American College of Rhuematology (ACR), 165

anatomy, *xi*, 1, 6, 10–17, 23, 113, 128, 169

anesthesia, 22

ankyloglossia. *See* tongue, -tied

antidepressants. *See* medications, antidepressants

anxiety, 22, 71, 105, 112, 118, 119, 125, 165, 199–203, 205. *See also* panic attacks; stress

appliance, mouth, 70, 74–76. *See also* splint

arthritis (also degeneration), *xi*, 4, 12–15, 20–22, 33, 68, 135, 149, 155, 166, 170, 174, 177, 180, 200; degenerative, 22, 33, 174; osteoarthritis, 4, 12, 13, 177; rheumatoid, 4

Arthritis Research Commission (ARC), 180

asthma, 109, 113, 118

aspartame, 187

asymmetry. *See* posture

B

back, *xii*, 33–35, 38–44, 48, 56–60, 65, 71, 190, 195, 218; pain, 2–3, 46–47, 61, 130, 132, 136–139, 162, 191, 200; supports, 8–9, 49–50, 54, 65, 71, 153, 222

bands (anterior and posterior), 5, 13–15, 30–31, 123, 169–182. *See also* ligaments

benign joint hypermobility syndrome. *See* hypermobility; syndromes, hypermobility and benign joint hypermobility (BJHS)

biofeedback, 24

bite, 17, 20–21, 67–76, 84, 143, 147; biting, 24; changes, 2–3, 5, 85, 93, 99, 120, 122; fingernails, 20, 147; guard, 218; line in mouth, 69; pain, 144–149. *See also* mouth guard; teeth

bones, 21, 36–46, 124, 146–150, 169–177, 199, 206–208, 226; hyoid, 86–87, 94, 152; mandible, 1, 10–14, 70, 76; mandibular condyle, 11–15, 30, 61, 68, 109, 170–175; pelvis, 34–38, 42, 47–48, 58, 60, 125, 138, 192; skull/

temporal bone, 1, 10–15, 17–18,
    96–97, 101, 136, 154–161, 189,
    192, 194; spurs, 12, 170
bottles, baby, 24, 88, 99
braces, 5, 21, 94. *See also* ortho-
    dontist
bracing of jaw muscles, 68–70,
    224. *See also* teeth, clenching
    and grinding
breathing, 7–8, 32, 59, 64, 105–118,
    193, 198–204, 212, 221, 223–227;
    belly (diaphragmatic), 42, 106,
    111, 150; chest (apical), 23, 80,
    88–89, 103, 110, 147, 153; mouth
    (nose), 20, 23, 80, 88–89, 103,
    110, 147, 153; rate, 108–109, 111–
    113; techniques, 73, 114–119, 147,
    233
bruxism. *See* teeth, grinding
    (bruxing)

C
caffeine, 26, 62, 70, 73, 82, 100, 125,
    187, 224
calcium, 27, 125, 204. *See* vitamins
    and minerals
calm (muscles and mind). *See* re-
    lax (relaxation)
capsule, capsulitis of temporo-
    mandibular joint, 14–15, 18, 21,
    148–149, 169, 178–179. *See also*
    synovial fluid
cartilage. *See* disk
causes: of disk displacement; of
    muscle pain; of teeth clenching;
    of temporomandibular joint
    disorders. *See* contributing fac-
    tors (possible causes)
central sensitivity syndrome
    (CSS). *See* nerves, central sen-

sitivity syndrome (CSS), hyper-
    irritable; syndromes, central
    sensitivity (CSS)
chemical(s), 186, 198; imbalance
    of, 106, 106, 204
cheese, 27, 187
chewing, 1–4, 14, 16–20, 24–28,
    67–68, 74, 83, 98, 100–102, 123,
    135, 144–147, 150, 168, 176, 183,
    185, 187, 193. *See also* swallow
chill stress. *See* cold, sensitivity
chocolate, 187
clenching. *See* teeth, clenching
clicking (jaw), 3–4, 77, 78, 172. *See
    also* disk, clicking
cognitive problems, 165
cold: ice/packs, 63, 100, 126, 190,
    193–196; sensitivity, 100, 126,
    143–144, 158, 160, 194; viral
    sickness, 109
computer: ergonomics, 8, 47–55,
    65, 137, 141, 156, 158, 160, 164,
    185–186, 197, 222, 230; glasses
    for, 43; as an irritant, 48, 62,
    125, 185, 207
connective tissue, 121, 131, 167, 179,
    190; of temporomandibular
    joint, 1, 15–18, 21, 182. *See also*
    bands; fascia; ligaments; tem-
    poromandibular joint
contributing factors (possible
    causes): of disk displacement,
    171–183; of muscle pain, 55,
    121–126, 131–134, 145, 149, 155,
    158, 167; of teeth clenching, 70;
    of temporomandibular joint
    disorders, *x–xiii*, 4–5, 14, 23,
    73, 121, 123; Cornell University
    Ergonomics. *See* computer,
    ergonomics

crepitus (crunch, gravel), 170. *See also* arthritis; degeneration
crying, 186

D
dairy foods, 112. *See also* cheese; diet; foods
degeneration/degenerative, 4, 13, 15, 20–21, 22. *See also* arthritis
dental, 226; American Dental Association ADA, 229; National Institute of Dental and Craniofascial Research (NIDCR), 230; procedures, 22, 80, 125, 144, 147, 176
depression, 32, 71, 105, 112, 125, 156, 165, 199–203, 206. *See also* medications, antidepressants (includes selective serotonin uptake inhibitors [SSRIs])
diabetes, 105
diaphragm, 42, 77, 80–81, 103, 106–110, 113–119, 142, 150, 201, 218, 221, 223. *See also* breathing, belly (diaphragmatic)
diary (headache or symptom), 6, 134, 184, 188–190, 196, 224
diet: allergies (food), 184, 187–190, 230; guidelines, 27; healthy, *xiii*, 25, 27, 72; soft-food, 25–26, 178
digastric. *See* muscles, digastric
disk: cervical, 61; jaw (also called meniscus, fibrocartilage pad), 13–18, 22, 31, 33, 36, 68, 120, 148–149, 169–183; clicking (also anterior disk dislocation with reduction), 75, 170–177; herniation of cervical, 33, 61; locking

(also anterior disk dislocation without reduction), 173–177
disorientation, 187
dizziness, 17, 33, 71, 112, 140, 153, 188
"double-jointed." *See* hypermobility; syndromes, hypermobility and benign joint hypermobility (BJHS)

E
ear: pain, 3, 132, 168; ringing, 3, 11, 33, 141, 146; stuffy/fullness, 11
ear, nose, and throat doctor (ENT), 118, 168. *See also* physician
Ehlers-Danlos syndrome. *See* syndromes, Ehlers-Danlos
ergonomic. *See* computer, ergonomics
exercise, *xii, xvi*, 10, 13, 18, 38, 42, 46–47, 53, 62–63, 74, 77, 106, 119, 124, 127, 129–130, 168, 175, 190, 191, 198–219; aerobic, 206–209, 211, 213, 215; anaerobic, 207–209; benefits, 205–206, 208; breathing, 111–119; Butterfly Stretch, 164; Calf Stretch, 216–217; Chin Tuck, 160–161; Crossover Arm Stretch, 138–139; Ear-to-Shoulder Stretch, 139–140; guidelines, 205, 208–209, 211, 218; Hamstring Stretch, 215–216; Hands-Behind-Back Stretch, 164–165; Hands-Behind-Head Stretch, 153–154; intensity, 211–213; Lopsided Blowfish, The, 148; Orbiting, 77–78, 148, 152, 178, 183, 192; Orbiting with Finger Lengthening of Tem-

ples, 145; precautions, *xvi*, 122, 135, 143, 167, 192, 209–210, 213; Quadriceps Stretch, 216–217; relaxation, 25, 73, 201–202; Relaxation Shoulder Rolls, 140, 163; Rolling Nod, The, 142–143; Rotation, Chin-to-Shoulder Head-Hang Stretch, 158–159; speech, 92–93, 103–104; Sitting Head-Hang Stretch, 156–157; stabilization, 179, 182, 214; Suboccipital Release, 161; swallowing, 94–98, 100–114; tongue, 84–92, 98, 104; Tongue Waggle, 150–152; upper lip, 79–82

F
fascia, 121
fatigue, 165; muscle or joint, 3, 24, 32, 68, 125, 179
fibromyalgia, 4, 120, 122, 126, 128, 135, 199, 208–209, 220, 230. *See also* syndromes, fibromyalgia; symptoms, fibromyalgia
first aid, 25, 188–197, 227
foods, 23, 25–28. *See also* diet: allergies (food); headache
frenulum, short. *See* tongue, -tied

G
gastrointestinal, 71, 199. *See also* syndromes, irritable bowel (and bladder)
genetics, 23
glasses (includes bifocals and trifocals), 17, 43, 51, 160, 186, 197
gout, 125
grinding. *See* teeth, grinding (bruxing)

gum, 4, 19, 24–25, 28, 135, 147, 150, 168, 213–214

H
habits, 7–8, 17–18, 19–20, 220–224. *See also* injury; posture; teeth, clenching
head, *xi–xii*, 2, 4–5, 10–11, 16–18, 20–22, 24–26, 40, 83–84, 87–88, 95–98, 100–102, 107, 115, 118, 124–125, 129–132, 134, 136, 138–139, 141–143, 153–165, 177, 199, 203, 206–207, 213; posture of, 30–66, 69–71, 77, 85, 109–110, 114, 122, 144, 147, 155, 158, 163, 191–192, 214
headache, *ii*, 2–5, 17, 21, 32, 38, 52, 68, 71, 88, 95, 100, 106, 109, 112, 119–120, 123–133, 140–143, 154, 158–159, 165, 167–168, 184–197, 199–200, 216, 218, 225–226, 230; diary, 188–189; migraine, 105–106, 140, 185; treatment, 189–195; triggers, 185–189, 230. *See also* diet, allergies; nerves, occipital
headset. *See* phone, headset
heart rate, 211–212
heat (pads, moist), 128–129, 189–197
heel lift, 37–38
hemipelvis, 37–38, 125, 138
hormones, 180, 184, 186, 198, 204
hygienist, dental, 20, 227
hyoid bone. *See* bones, hyoid
hypermobility (of joints), 16, 41, 179–183. *See also* syndromes, hypermobility and benign joint hypermobility (BJHS)

hypersensitivity, 17, 106, 127–128, jaw and teeth, 143; lights, sounds, smells, and pain, 199; nipple, 162; 180, 182. *See* nerves, hyperirritable; nervous system, hyper- or oversensitive; syndromes, central sensitivity (CSS)

hypoglycemia, 125

I

ice, 4, 17, 19, 25, 26, 28, 100, 129, 147, 150, 155, 189, 190, 192–194, 197

immobilize, 130, 147

infection(s), 3, 23, 126, 142, 147, 151, 183, 200, 225, 227

inflammation, 15, 76, 129, 190, 193, 195

injury, 21–27, 121–122, 130–131, 134, 191–193, 207–208, 213, 228; prevention by stretching, 213–215; whiplash, 16–17, 22, 120, 138, 141, 153, 155, 158, 173, 178, 180

irritable bowel syndrome (IBS). *See* syndromes, irritable bowel (and bladder)

J

jaw, lower. *See* mandible

jaw, joint. *See* temporomandibular joint (TMJ)

jaw, joint capsule. *See* capsule, capsulitis of temporomandibular joint

joint, hypermobility. *See* hypermobility; syndromes, hypermobility and benign joint hypermobility (BJHS)

L

lateral pterygoid. *See* muscles, lateral pterygoid, medial pterygoid

leg-length discrepancy, 35–38, 64–65, 125, 138, 142, 149, 179 also ligamentous laxity . See hypermobility (of joints)

lips, 17–18, 23, 67, 76–82, 87–89, 91, 94, 96–100, 109–111, 114, 116, 119, 147, 149, 193, 195, 218, 221, 223; bite, 20; chapped, 109, 111; exercises, 79–81, 91, 93; licking, 24; short or tight upper lip, 76–79– 82, 88–99, 101, 109–110, 119, 224

ligaments, 1, 5, 15, 16, 18, 21–22, 30, 31–32, 38, 41, 94, 169–183, 205. *See also* bands; hypermobility; whiplash

locking jaw joint. *See* disk, locking

lungs, 106–110, 114–115, 205, 207

M

macroglossia. *See* tongue, large

mandible, 1, 10–15, 18, 31, 43, 64, 146, 149, 151, 169, 170; condyle, 11–15, 30, 61, 68, 170–175; coronoid process, 143; fossa, 11; resting position of, 84–88. *See also* temporomandibular joint

manipulation, 46, 192. *See also* mobilization

manual techniques, 38, 89, 129, 160, 161, 190, 192. *See also* manipulation; mobilization

Marfan syndrome. *See* syndromes, Marfan

massage, 114, 127–129, 138, 191, 219

masseter. *See* muscles, masseter

maxilla (upper jaw), 146, 149
mastication, muscles of, 16. *See also* chewing
medial pterygoid. *See* muscles, medial pterygoid
medications (also pills), 81, 184, 186, 188; antidepressants (includes selective serotonin reuptake inhibitors, SSRIs), 70–72, 81–82; for asthma, 113; painkiller, 4, 188, 203; with ultrasound, 129
memory, 165, 187, 200, 221
meningitis, signs of, 191
meniscus. *See* disk
menopause, 186
menstruation, 180, 186. *See also* hormones
menu planning, 25, 27, 224
metabolic(ism) deficiencies, 125, 167–168; pump, 15; or TMJ, 31
minerals. *See* vitamins and minerals
mobilization, 191. *See also* exercises; manipulation
mouse, computer. *See* computer, ergonomics
mouth, 10, 20, 25, 43, 69–74, 76–82, 86, 88–89, 91–104, 114, 116, 127, 129, 145, 147, 150, 175, 218, 223, 226; breathing, 20, 23, 64, 76, 80, 84, 88–90, 100, 109–111, 118, 119, 142, 144, 147, 153, 227–228; development of, 84, 118; difficulty opening/closing, 3, 15, 68, 78, 143–146, 152–153, 170, 171–175, 214; dry (xerostomia), 70, 73; guard, 25, 70, 74, 228; how far to open, 174–178, 195; overopening or prolonged opening, 16, 32, 174–176, 182–183; pain, 151–152; sores, 126. *See also* appliance, mouth; palate; splint

mouth guard, 25, 70, 74, 218, 228. *See also* appliance, mouth; splint
MSG, 187
muscles, 1, 16–18, 30, 41, 43, 72, 120–168, 176, 182, 192, 198, 205, 207, 208–210; abdominal, 38, 42, 110, 114, 116, 131; balance, 32, 36, 38, 42–43, 120, 177–179, 192, 225; calf, 42, 216–217; calm/relax, 18, 23, 32, 50, 58, 72–76, 77–82, 134–135, 176; digastric, 132, 152–154; hamstrings, 41–42, 47, 214–216; lateral pterygoid, 14–16, 31, 132, 148–151, 168–170, 178; masseter, 16, 132, 146–148, 151, 153, 168; mastication, 16, 68–76, 185; medial pterygoid, 16, 132, 149, 151–152, 168; mentalis, 79; neck, middle and deep/semi-spinalis, mulitifidi, rotators, 132, 154; pain, 3, 12, 21, 27, 32, 33, 61, 67–68, 120–168, 171–172; neck, 50, 59, 61, 94–98, 100–104, 107–109, 115, 116, 119, 184, 190–192, 218, 223; palpation of, 133; pectoralis, 43, 132, 138, 156, 162–164, 185, 218; posterior cervical, 132, 155–157; quadriceps, 42, 134, 215–217; spasm of, 15, 31, 121, 122, 126, 130, 178, 193, 195; splenius, 132, 157–159; sternocleidomastoid (SCM), 132, 140–142, 147; suboccipitals,

132, 159–161; techniques, 38, 128–129, 131, 190, 192–195; temporalis, 16, 132, 133, 143–145; tension/strain, 26, 30, 32, 44, 53, 59, 68–71, 94, 103, 106, 118, 120, 134, 178, 179, 185–186, 193, 195, 198–202, 204, 221, 223–224; tongue, 83; trapezius, 32, 43, 132, 135–139, 140, 145, 147, 154, 157, 168. *See also* diaphragm; stretch(es); trigger points

muscle energy techniques, 38, 129

music, 28, 117, 202

musicians, 24, 28, 158

myofascial pain syndrome, *xv*, 120–167, 199, 207–208. *See also* syndromes, myofascial pain

N

National Headache Association, 187, 230

National Institute of Dental and Craniofascial Research, 2, 230

National Institutes of Health (NIH), 2, 3, 27, 72, 109, 172, 187, 230

National Institute of Neurological Disorders and Stroke, 185

National TMJ Association, *xvi*

nausea, 25, 33, 277, 187, 191

neck, *xii*, 2, 16, 18, 20–23, 30, 34, 38–39, 42, 44, 46, 48, 50, 55, 65–66, 77, 83–84, 88, 122–124, 126–128, 131, 135–137, 141–142, 154–167, 195–197, 205–206, 209–210, 218, 225–228; artery, 143, 192; breathing, 107–109, 114–119, 223; disc herniation, 33; exercises, 142; long, 154;

pain, *xi–xii*, 2–5, 17, 21, 25–28, 30, 32–33, 44, 46, 48, 50–53, 55, 59, 88, 109, 120, 130, 132, 136–137, 140–141, 154–155, 157–158, 167, 184–185, 189, 190–193, 196–197, 199–200, 216, 218; stiff, 187; stretch, 139–140, 153–154, 156–157, 164, 213–214

nerves, 18, 21, 48, 78, 122–123; breathing to calm, 113; central sensitivity syndrome (CSS), 17, 199; cranial, 17; entrapped/pinched/irritated, 122, 123, 126, 186; hyperirritable, 106, 113, 122; occipital, 17, 154–155, 189; signs of involvement, 191; trigeminal, 17

nervous system, 17; autonomic, 17, 198; central, 17, 73, 150, 199; hyper- or oversensitive, 165, 198–205; sympathetic, 108

neuralgia. *See* nerves, occipital, trigeminal

NIH. *See* National Institutes of Health

nitrates/nitrites, 187

nose, stuffy, 64, 89

numbness, 187, 191

nutritional inadequacies, 27, 124, 125, 168. *See also* diet, healthy; vitamins and minerals

nuts, 26, 147, 187

O

obsessive-compulsive disorder, 71

occipital neuralgia. *See* nerves, occipital

Orbiting. *See* exercises, Orbiting

orofacial pain. *See* temporomandibular joint disorders
orthodontist, 93–94, 225. *See also*
braces
osteogenesis imperfecta, 180
osteoporosis, 13, 40, 199, 204

P

pacifiers, 20, 23, 24, 85, 88, 99,
227
pain, 73; chronic, *xi*, 55, 64, 106,
135, 199, 213, 229. *See* back, pain;
headache; myofascial pain syndrome; neck, pain; syndromes,
chronic pain; trigger points
painkillers. *See* medications, painkiller
palate, 76, 86–88, 99; alveolar
ridge, 86, 93, 96–97; development, 84; exercises, 91, 93, 99;
high, 89–90; rugae, 86; swallowing, 102; and thumb sucking, 23, 85, 88, 90, 99
panic attacks, 112. *See also* anxiety
parafunctional (activities or habits), 20, 23
parasympathetic nervous system.
See nervous system, sympathetic
pectoralis. *See* muscles, pectoralis
pelvis. *See* bones, pelvis
perceived exertion scale, 212–213
perfectionism, 112
perfume/fragrance, 186
phone, 4, 28, 51, 125, 138, 141, 186,
189, 222; books, 47, 53, 66;
headset, 24, 28, 138, 141, 222;
speaker, 24, 28, 51, 138, 141, 222
physical therapy (PT), *xiii*, *xv*, 21,
31, 55, 73–74, 177–178, 184, 201,
225, 229
physician (doctor), *x*, *xiii*, *xv*, *xvi*,
6, 12, 27, 43, 56, 59, 63, 72, 80–
82, 90, 102, 109, 110, 112, 113, 116,
118, 123, 125, 129, 130, 153, 167,
168, 177, 183, 187, 190–191, 194,
206, 208–210, 213, 219, 225, 227;
allergist, 118; choosing a, 204;
ear, nose, and throat (ENT),
118–119, 168
pillows, 8–9, 38, 48, 50–51, 55, 58–
63, 65–66, 71, 124, 137, 142, 155,
158–159, 163, 196, 222; picking/
choosing, 56–58
post-traumatic stress disorder
(PTSD), 71, 202
posture, 7, 28, 29–66, 70, 77, 84,
96, 97, 99, 102–103, 149, 190,
196, 199, 202–203, 221–227; bal-
anced/neutral/healthy, 8–18,
29–30, 54–66, 94, 100, 114,
116, 119, 168; exercises/"quick
fix," 46, 160, 161, 163–165, 195,
210, 214, 218–219; forward
head/slouched, 17, 29–31, 43,
69–70, 85, 110, 144, 147, 155, 163,
185–186; how to assess, 33–40;
sitting, 47, 54, 65–66, 71, 168;
sleep, 29, 55–63, 65, 71, 82, 102,
144–149, 163; standing, 40–47,
65–66, 71, 168; symptoms of
poor, 33; unbalanced, 22, 24,
31–33, 51–56, 85, 94–85, 100,
110, 125, 160, 179. *See also* leg-
length discrepancy; scoliosis
PoTSB TLC, 17–18, 29, 67, 72, 74,
77, 82, 84, 93, 103–104, 105, 113,
119, 183, 192, 195, 221–222

pterygoid. *See* muscles, lateral
　　pterygoid, medial pterygoid

R

reading in bed, 63; sitting 49
relax (relaxation), 18, 25, 30, 32, 33,
　　43, 48, 50, 52, 54, 60, 62, 69–78,
　　81–82, 86–88, 91, 98, 100, 107,
　　108, 112–116, 118, 129, 131, 134,
　　135, 138, 140, 142, 144, 145, 147,
　　148, 150, 151, 153, 156, 158, 160,
　　163, 172, 178, 180, 192–195, 201–
　　202, 204, 218, 219, 221, 223
restless leg syndrome. *See* syn-
　　dromes, restless leg
ringing. *See* ear, ringing

S

scoliosis, 38–40, 44, 167
selective serotonin reuptake in-
　　hibitors (SSRIs). *See* medica-
　　tions, antidepressants (includes
　　selective serotonin reuptake
　　inhibitors [SSRIs])
sewing, 155
shoulder(s), 4, 24, 33–37, 39, 42–
　　47, 50–53, 56, 58–61, 65, 110,
　　115–116, 123, 124, 136–143, 154–
　　159, 162–164, 175, 185–187, 218,
　　222; pain, 2, 3, 46, 126, 130–132,
　　162, 191
shoulder blades (scapula), 34, 43,
　　137, 164
sinuses (blockage, infection,
　　open), 64, 118, 140, 186, 227
sippee cups, 24, 99
skull. *See* bones, skull
sleep, 1, 9, 18, 29, 55–65, 81, 93,
　　101–102, 125, 168, 184, 188, 190;
　　apnea, 33, 64, 70, 73, 80, 90,

109, 225; disorders, 23, 26, 70,
　　90, 109, 186, 199, 200–203, 229;
　　healthy, 8, 55–63, 70–71, 126,
　　142, 156, 205; positions/posture,
　　8, 9, 22, 24, 29–30, 32, 33, 37, 43,
　　55–62, 65, 68, 70–71, 72, 82, 102,
　　109, 124–125, 144, 149, 151, 158,
　　160, 163, 168, 177, 183, 185, 186,
　　195, 227; sleep specialist, 56, 63,
　　125, 225, 229. *See also* posture,
　　sleep
slouch. *See* muscles, pectoralis;
　　posture, forward head, unbal-
　　anced
smoking (includes nicotine and
　　tobacco), 24, 70, 73, 125, 203
spasm of muscles, 15, 31, 121, 122,
　　126, 130, 178, 193, 195. *See also*
　　muscles
speech, 81, 90, 104, 187; exercises,
　　85, 92–93; therapy/speech
　　language pathologist, *xv*, 85,
　　88, 90, 93, 94, 99, 103, 104, 225,
　　229–230
splenius. *See* muscles, splenius
splint (occlusal), 74–76, 81–82, 144,
　　147, 149, 151, 168, 177, 178, 224.
　　See also appliance, mouth; splint
　　"Spot, The." *See* palate, alveolar
　　ridge
spray and stretch technique,
　　128–129
SSRIs. *See* medications, antide-
　　pressants (includes selective
　　serotonin uptake inhibitors
　　[SSRIs])
stabilization. *See* exercise, stabili-
　　zation
sternocleidomastoid (SCM). *See*
　　muscles, sternocleidomastoid

stress, 4, 72–73, 108–109, 111, 188, 198–206, 218–219; emotional, *x*, 4, 17, 22, 69, 71–73, 89, 108–109, 111–113, 116, 118, 135, 147, 150–151, 179, 186, 189, 198–206, 218–219; management, 73, 114–118, 119, 200–206, 211, 219, 224; physical/mechanical, 13–14, 20, 24–28, 32, 55, 71–73, 83, 100, 120, 122, 124, 126, 137, 147, 151, 153, 176, 179, 186. *See also* anxiety; relax (relaxation)

stretch(es), *xvi*, 32, 38, 42–43, 48, 55, 102, 122–135, 180, 201, 207, 209, 213, 224; Butterfly Stretch, 164; Calf Stretch, 216–217; Chin Tuck, 160–161; Crossover Arm Stretch, 138–139; diaphragm, 115–117; Ear-to-Shoulder Stretch, 139–140; frenulum of tongue, 29–91; guidelines, 48, 51, 53–54, 122–135, 190–197, 218–219, 214–215; Hamstring Stretch, 215–216; Hands-Behind-Back Stretch, 164–165; Hands-Behind-Head Stretch, 153–154; Lopsided Blowfish, The, 148; Orbiting, 77–78, 148, 152, 178, 183, 192; Orbiting with Finger Lengthening of Temples, 145; Quadriceps Stretch, 216–217; Relaxation Shoulder Rolls, 140, 163; Rolling Nod, 142–143; Rotation Chin-to-Shoulder Head-Hang Stretch, 158–159; Sitting Head-Hang Stretch, 156–157; Suboccipital Release, 161; Tongue Waggle, 150–152; upper lip, 79–82, 89, 119, 224

subconscious. *See* habits

supplements. *See* diet; vitamins and minerals

surgery, 5, 15, 59, 106, 174, 176, 177, 225

swallow, 1, 7, 9, 16–18, 22, 23, 32, 58, 60, 81, 83–104, 147, 153, 185, 193, 195, 220–223; development, 98–100, 227; difficulty, 3, 225; exercises, 100–104, 228; get help, 225; how to, 67, 96–98

sympathetic nervous system. *See* nervous system

symptom diary. *See* diary (headache or symptom)

symptoms: concerning, 187–191; depression, 156; fibromyalgia, 164–166; increase in, 80; of occipital neuralgia, 17; poor posture, 33, 47–48; onset of TMJ, 21, 200; temporomandibular joint disorders (TMJ), *xi*, *xiii*, 1–7, 9, 11, 16, 21, 23, 75, 85, 117, 133–167, 172, 174, 186, 199, 200, 203, 209–210, 220–221. *See also* asthma

syndromes (and inherited disorders): central sensitivity (CSS), 17; chronic pain, *xi*, 55, 64, 106, 135, 199, 213, 229; Ehlers-Danlos, 180; fibromyalgia, 4, 120, 122, 126, 128, 135, 199, 208–209, 220; hypermobility and benign joint hypermobility (BJHS), 17, 106, 127–128, 180, 182, 199; hyperventilation, 105; irritable bowel (and bladder), 165, 199; Marfan, 180, myofascial pain, *xv*, 120–167, 199, 207–208; osteogenesis imperfecta, 180;

restless leg, 72, 165; Reynaud's, 194. *See also* hypermobility (of joints)

synovial fluid, 14–15, 18, 68, 172

T

Tai Chi, 201

teeth, 7, 22–26, 67–82, 83–88, 90, 93, 104, 114, 116, 171, 172, 174, 176, 178, 223, 226; apart, 18, 23, 43, 67–82, 147, 149, 193, 195, 221, 223; clenching, 3, 4, 15, 19–20, 23, 43–44, 58, 60, 68–82, 94, 125, 147, 186, 218; grinding (bruxing), 3, 19–20, 23, 58, 68–82, 104, 144, 147, 150–153, 168, 199; speech, 85–87, 92, 103, 104, 110, 223; when swallowing, 94–96, 98–102, 110. *See also* appliances; bracing of jaw muscles; medications, antidepressants (includes selective serotonin reuptake inhibitors, SSRIs); splint; stress

television, 50, 52, 63, 190, 196

temporal bone, 10–15, 18, 170–174; articular tubercle, 11; auditory meatus (ear), 11

temporalis. *See* muscles, temporalis

temporomandibular joint (TMJ), 1–3, 18, 23, 32, 149, 172, 182–183, 194; anatomy, 10–11, 12–16, 169–171, 182; expert, 225–226; protection, 23–28, 58–61, 70–73, 77–78, 81, 86–89, 99–100, 168, 182–183, 220

temporomandibular joint disorder (TMD), *xvi*, 15–17, 20–27, 31, 67–70, 94, 120, 128, 131, 132, 146, 148–152, 164, 168, 172, 174, 180, 190, 198–199, 203, 226–228 therapy. *See* physical therapy; speech therapy

throat, 96, 102, 118, 176; pain, 132, 141, 151

thumb sucking, 23, 85, 88, 90, 99

thyroid, 125–126, 147, 167

tingling, 191

tinnitus. *See* ear, ringing

tissue, connective. *See* bands; ligaments; muscles

tongue, 18, 69, 81–82, 83–104, 109; anatomy, 87; exercises/training, 76–78, 91–93, 144, 145, 150–152, 178, 228; large (macroglossia), 90; position, 7, 9, 22, 43, 70–72, 84–88, 110, 114, 116, 119, 147, 193, 195, 221, 223, 227; rule of, 175–176; thrust, *xv*, 5, 32, 83–85, 99–100, 184, 223, 225; -tied (ankyloglossia), 86, 89–90

tooth ache/pain, 3, 120, 122–123, 132–133, 142, 143, 146, 151, 152; infection, 144, 147. *See* teeth, clenching, grinding (bruxing)

trapezius. *See* muscles, trapezius

trauma. *See* injury; whiplash

trigeminal nerve. *See* nerves, trigeminal

trigger points, 59, 122–135, 167–168, 179, 185, 191–193, 195–196, 199; causes, 124–126, 179; cycle diagram, 121; muscle groups: digastric, 132, 152–154; lateral pterygoid, 132, 148–150; masseter, 132, 146–148; medial pterygoid, 132, 149, 151–152; neck middle and deep/semispi-

nalis, mulitifidi, rotators, 132, 154, pectoralis, 132, 162–164; posterior cervical, 132, 155–157; splenius, 132, 157–159; sterno-cleidomastoid (SCM), 132, 140–142, 147; suboccipitals, 132, 159–161; temporalis, 132, 143–145; trapezius, 132, 136–139, 147; treatment, 126–135, 195–196, 214, 229. *See also* under each muscle group
tumors, 187

V

vision 63, 226; blurred/change, 17, 33, 141, 158, 187. *See also* glasses
vitamins and minerals, 27, 125, 147, 150, 204. *See also* diet; nutritional inadequacies
vomiting, 22, 25, 125, 176, 187, 191

W

walk, walking, 30, 36, 38, 42, 46–52, 98, 108, 134, 177, 201, 207–209, 213, 215, 219, 222. *See also* exercise, aerobic
weakness, 43, 124, 191
weather, 126, 187
whiplash, 16–17, 22, 120, 138, 141, 153, 155, 158, 173, 178, 180.
Wolff's Law, 12
writing, 51, 55, 155, 204

X

xerostomia. *See* mouth, dry

Y

yawning, 3, 23, 175–176, 178, 180, 183. *See also* mouth, overopening
yoga, 113, 201, 207, 219

POSITIVE OPTIONS FOR CROHN'S DISEASE by *Joan Gomez, M.D.*

Crohn's disease is an inflammatory bowel condition that, while non-fatal, can be devastating. This book discusses who is at risk and why, and addresses what can be done, including self-care.

192 pages ... 1 illus. ... Paperback $13.95

POSITIVE OPTIONS FOR LIVING WITH YOUR OSTOMY
by *Dr. Craig A. White*

This book is a complete, supportive guide to dealing with the practical and emotional aspects of life after ostomy surgery.

144 pages ... 4 illus. ... Paperback $12.95

POSITIVE OPTIONS FOR HIATUS HERNIA by *Tom Smith, M.D.*

A hiatus hernia is a common, potentially serious condition that occurs when the upper part of the stomach pushes through the diaphragm. This book describes tests, treatments, and self-help options.

128 pages ... 4 illus. ... 2 tables ... Paperback $12.95

POSITIVE OPTIONS FOR COLORECTAL CANCER
by *Carol Ann Larson*

Colorectal cancer, the second leading cancer killer of adults in the U.S., is treatable if caught in time. This book tells you everything you need to know about prevention, diagnosis, and treatment.

168 pages ... 10 illus. ... Paperback $12.95

POSITIVE OPTIONS FOR REFLEX SYMPATHETIC DYSTROPHY (RSD) by *Elena Juris*

RSD, also called Complex Regional Pain Syndrome, is characterized by severe nerve pain and extreme sensitivity to touch. This book covers medical information, practical advice, and holistic therapies.

224 pages ... 2 illus. ... Paperback $14.95

POSITIVE OPTIONS FOR ANTIPHOSPHOLIPID SYNDROME (APS)
by *Triona Holden*

Also called Hughes syndrome and "sticky blood," APS is implicated in many serious health problems. This book identifies the symptoms and provides important information on diagnosis and treatment.

144 pages ... Paperback $12.95

POSITIVE OPTIONS FOR SEASONAL AFFECTIVE DISORDER (SAD)
by *Fiona Marshall and Peter Cheevers*

About 10 million Americans suffer from SAD. This book helps distinguish the condition from classic depression and chronic fatigue, and suggests ways to alleviate the symptoms and live optimally.

144 pages ... Paperback $13.95

Hunter House
FITNESS & BODY CARE

TREAT YOUR OWN KNEES by Jim Johnson, P.T.

An inexpensive, compact, useful book. Simple illustrations depict the muscles responsible for knee pain and the correct way to perform exercises that can enhance knee strength, flexibility, and endurance.
128 pages ... 21 illus. ... Paperback $10.95

TREAT YOUR BACK WITHOUT SURGERY: The Best Nonsurgical Alternatives for Eliminating Back and Neck Pain
by Stephen Hochschuler, M.D., and Bob Reznik, MBA *... 2nd Edition*

Clear discussion of nonsurgical techniques from Tai Chi and massage to chiropractic and acupuncture. Includes exercise plans, information on diet and stress management, and tips to ease everyday pain.
224 pages ... 58 b/w photos ... 6 illus. ... Paperback $17.95

THE CHIROPRACTOR'S SELF-HELP BACK AND BODY BOOK: How You Can Relieve Common Aches and Pains at Home and on the Job by Samuel Homola, D.C.

Home help for people with chronic head, neck, arm, wrist, back, hip, leg, and shoulder pain. Includes information on handling arthritis, protecting a weak back, and shopping for good chiropractic care.
320 pages ... 42 illus. ... Paperback $19.95

SHAPEWALKING: Six Easy Steps to Your Best Body
by Marilyn Bach, Ph.D., and Lorie Schleck, M.A., P.T. *... 2nd Edition*

ShapeWalking is a low-cost walking-cum-fitness program that includes aerobic exercise, strength training, and flexibility stretching. Ideal for people who want to control weight, develop muscle definition, prevent or reverse loss of bone density, and do spot-shaping.
144 pages ... 73 photos ... 9 illus. ... Paperback $14.95

THE GOOD FOOT BOOK: A Guide for Men, Women, Children, Athletes, Seniors — Everyone by Glenn Copeland with Stan Solomon

From a leading podiatrist: advice on prevention and cures for common foot problems like bunions, hammer toes, corns, calluses, and warts, as well as the special foot problems of seniors and athletes.
240 pages ... 42 illus. ... Paperback $17.95

GET FIT WHILE YOU SIT: Easy Workouts from Your Chair
by Charlene Torkelson

Written for office workers, travelers, and those with movement limitations or special conditions. Includes a low-impact One-Hour Chair Program, five compact workouts, and the Ten-Minute Miracles: easy-to-remember exercises perfect for when you are at work or traveling.
160 pages ... 210 photos ... Paperback $16.95 ... Spiral bound $21.95